MW01235945

OMNI DIET

HEALTH REVOLUTION
SUCCESS PLANNER

**The Revolutionary
70% PLANT + 30% PROTEIN
Program to Lose Weight, Reverse
Disease, Fight Inflammation, and
CHANGE YOUR LIFE FOREVER**

TANA AMEN, B.S.N., R.N.

"The Omni Diet is a thoughtful, practical approach to eating.
Discover delicious, wholesome food that benefits your health for good."
Mehmet Oz, M.D.

BOOKS BY TANA AMEN , B.S.N., R.N.

Change Your Brain, Change Your Body Cookbook

Eat Healthy with the Brain Doctor's Wife Cookbook

Get Healthy with the Brain Doctor's Wife Coaching Guide

MEDICAL DISCLAIMER

The information presented in this book is the result of years of practical experience and clinical research by the author. The information in this book, by necessity, is of a general nature and not a substitute for an evaluation or treatment by a competent medical specialist. If you believe you are in need of medical interventions please see a medical practitioner as soon as possible. The stories in this book are true. The names and circumstances of the stories have been changed to protect the anonymity of patients.

INTRODUCTION

[Create Your Personal Omni Health Revolution]

HOW TO USE THIS JOURNAL

The food you eat every day is either medicine that is helping you or it is literally making you sick and possibly shortening your life. By taking the necessary steps to put the Omni Diet into practice, you are taking back control over your body and your life. Congratulations for becoming a WARRIOR for your health.

I designed this daily journal to help you stay motivated and on track toward achieving all your goals. It is divided into six sections, with two weeks in each of the three phases that I outline in *The Omni Diet*. Each weekly section provides a brief summary of the highlighted step for that week that will help you lose excess weight, improve your energy, have better digestion, have glowing skin, and exude radiant health. Your journal is set up so that you can easily plan your Omni Diet meals for the next day. I find this to be invaluable for sticking with the program. As I always say, "If you fail to plan, you plan to fail." You will also find tips to motivate you and help you stick with your plan.

Each day also includes a checklist of healthy behaviors for you to choose from in order to help you achieve your desired goals. Imagine the satisfaction you'll feel as you accomplish your daily goals. Among the items on your list you will find:

- Your specific goal for the day

- Physical exercise

- Listing three things you're grateful for

- Drinking your full allotment of water (staying hydrated is crucial)

- Eating your veggies!

- Reaching out to others who support your goals

By taking just a few minutes each day to work with this journal, you will be making the habit of healthy living integral to your everyday life. It will keep your goals clearly before you, giving you the motivation to keep going, and the strength to make the choices that keep you feeling and looking your best.

This journal will be your companion for six weeks. But that is just the beginning. By the end of that time, you should be seeing the benefits of your healthy new lifestyle and you'll be eager to continue with it. Your tastes will change. You'll have a new relationship with the food you eat. And you'll have new enthusiasm for the beautiful possibilities of your life.

Know Your Important Numbers

As my husband, Dr. Amen says, "You cannot change what you do not measure!" As you get ready to start the Omni Diet, it is important to make a record of your current physical condition and habits. Then, at the end of the 6 weeks (some people prefer to check again after 12 weeks instead), check these numbers again to see how much progress you have made.

1. Body Mass Index (BMI):

Week 1   Week 6

Find your height in the left column, and then read across that row to find your weight. Your BMI is at the top of that column.

Underweight: Under 19
Normal weight: 19-24.9
Overweight: 25-29.9

Obese: 30 or higher
Morbid Obesity: 40 or higher

BODY MASS INDEX
BODY WEIGHT (IN POUNDS)

Height	20	21	22	23	24	25	26	27	28	29	30	35	40
4'10"	96	100	105	110	115	119	124	129	134	138	143	167	191
4'11"	99	104	109	114	119	124	128	133	138	143	148	173	198
5'0"	102	107	112	118	123	128	133	138	143	148	153	179	204
5'1"	106	111	116	122	127	132	137	143	148	153	158	185	211
5'2"	109	115	120	126	131	136	142	147	153	158	164	191	218
5'3"	113	118	124	130	135	141	146	152	158	163	169	197	225
5'4"	116	122	128	134	140	145	151	157	163	169	174	204	232
5'5"	120	126	132	138	144	150	156	162	168	174	180	210	240
5'6"	124	130	136	142	148	155	161	167	173	179	186	216	247
5'7"	127	134	140	146	153	159	166	172	178	185	191	223	255
5'8"	131	138	144	151	158	164	171	177	184	190	197	230	262
5'9"	135	142	149	155	162	169	176	182	189	196	203	236	270
5'10"	139	146	153	160	167	174	181	188	195	202	207	243	278
5'11"	143	150	157	165	172	179	186	193	200	208	215	250	286
6'0"	147	154	162	169	177	184	191	199	206	213	221	258	294
6'1"	151	159	166	174	182	189	197	204	212	219	227	265	302
6'2"	155	163	171	179	186	194	202	210	218	225	233	272	311
6'3"	160	168	176	184	192	200	208	216	224	232	240	279	319
6'4"	164	172	180	189	197	205	213	221	230	238	246	287	328

[CONTENTS]

Introduction: Create Your Personal Omni Health Revolution   1

Know Your Important Numbers   2

PHASE ONE

WEEK ONE

Jump The Canyon: The Gradual Process is of No Use At All   7

Exercise: Discover a New World of Food   9

Phase One-Week One Summary   26

WEEK TWO

Jump the Canyon: How to Stay on the Other Side   27

Exercise: Refine and Personalize Your Omni Diet   29

Phase One-Week Two Summary   46

PHASE TWO

WEEK ONE

Pump It Up: Stay on Track With a Food Journal   47

Exercise: Start Your Food Journal   49

Phase Two-Week One Summary   66

WEEK TWO

Pump It Up: Get Your Body Moving   67

Exercise: Follow Your Exercise Program   69

Phase Two-Week Two Summary   86

PHASE THREE

WEEK ONE

Relax Your Way to Better Health: Make 90/10 Your Golden Rule   87

Exercise: A Plan to Overcome Temptation   89

Phase Three-Week One Summary   106

WEEK TWO

Relax Your Way to Better Health: Better Sleep and Less Stress   107

Exercise: Steps to Improve Sleep and Reduce Stress   109

Phase Three-Week Two Summary   126

THE
OMNI
DIET

EXERCISE PLANNER

**The Revolutionary
70% PLANT + 30% PROTEIN
Program to Lose Weight, Reverse
Disease, Fight Inflammation, and
CHANGE YOUR LIFE FOREVER**

TANA AMEN, B.S.N., R.N.

"The Omni Diet is a thoughtful, practical approach to eating.
Discover delicious, wholesome food that benefits your health for good."

Mehmet Oz, M.D.

2. Current weight:

Week 1	Week 6

3. Desired weight:

Week 1	Week 6

4. Waist to Height Ratio:

Week 1	Week 6

Measure at your belly button with a tape measure. To be healthy, your waist size should be half your height or less in inches. Healthy ratio: Less than or equal to .5.

5. Number of Hours You Sleep at Night:

Week 1	Week 6

Blood Tests: Ask your doctor to order, or you can order them yourself by going to www.saveonlabs.com.

6. Vitamin D level:
Low: Below 30mg/dL   Optimal: 50-90mg/dL   High: Above 90mg/dL

Week 1	Week 6

7. Thyroid:

Thyroid-stimulating hormone (TSH) Healthy is below 2.5ulU/mL	Week 1	Week 6
Free T3 Healthy between 230 to 619 pg/dL	Week 1	Week 6
Free T4 Healthy between 0.7 to 1.9 ng/dL	Week 1	Week 6

8. C-reactive protein: Healthy range: 0.0 - 1.0mg/dL

Week 1	Week 6

9. Homocysteine: Healthy level: less than 10mmol/L (micromoles per liter)

Week 1	Week 6

10. HgA1C: Normal: 4.0 – 5.7   Elevated: over 5.7

Week 1	Week 6

11. Fasting blood sugar:
Normal: 70-90 mg/dL   Pre-diabetes: 91-125 mg/dL   Diabetes: 126 mg/dL or higher

Week 1	Week 6

12. Total Cholesterol:
Normal: 135-200 mg/dL, below 135 has been associated with depression.
HDL (>= 60 mg/dL)   LDL (<100 mg/dL) Triglycerides (<100 mg/dl)

Week 1   Week 6

13. Blood Pressure: Optimal: Less than 120/80

Week 1   Week 6

14. Ferritin: Total cholesterol: Ideal level for women: 15-200ng/mL

Week 1   Week 6

15. Free & Total Serum Testosterone:
Normal levels for women:
Free testosterone: 0.4-1.9 ng/dL   Total testosterone: 30-95 ng/dL

Week 1   Week 6

16. Cortisol: Total cholesterol Optimal: 11–14 µg/dL

Week 1   Week 6

17. DHEA-S: Total cholesterol Normal: 44–332 µg/dL

Week 1   Week 6

Know how many of the 12 most common preventable causes of death you have...then decrease them

Check all that apply. Use the first box for Week 1, the second box for Week 6.

☐ ☐ Smoking   ☐ ☐ High blood pressure

☐ ☐ BMI overweight/obese   ☐ ☐ Physical inactivity

☐ ☐ High fasting blood glucose   ☐ ☐ High LDL cholesterol

☐ ☐ Alcohol abuse   ☐ ☐ Low omega-3 fatty acids

☐ ☐ High processed/trans fat intake ☐ ☐ Low polyunsaturated fat intake

☐ ☐ High dietary salt

☐ ☐ Low intake of fruits and vegetables

Total: Week 1   Week 6

SUMMARY OF MY IMPORTANT NUMBERS

	Week 1	Week 6	Better? Yes/No
BMI			
Current Weight			
Weight to Height Ration			
Number of Days Slept 7 or More Hours			
Vitamin D			
TSH			
C-Reactive Protein			
Homocysteine			
HgAIC			
Fasting Blood Sugar			
Total Cholesterol			
Blood Pressure			
Ferritin			
Free Testosterone			
Total Testosterone			
Cortisol			
DHEA-S			
Total Number of Preventable Risk Factors			

Jump The Canyon

"THE GRADUAL PROCESS IS OF NO USE AT ALL."
– C.S. LEWIS

I've never been a believer in taking baby steps. You have to shut one door before another one opens. And that's especially true when it comes to adopting a healthy way of eating. That's because the components of the typical American diet have addictive qualities to them. As long as you continue to eat any of those foods, even in smaller quantities, you will be keeping your addictions to sugar and simple carbohydrates alive.

Going "cold turkey" isn't as hard as it sounds when you have a plan for replacing all those familiar energy-zapping, fat-laden foods, with fresh, satisfying, yummy foods that taste great and make you look and feel great. Eating a balanced 70 percent plant/30 percent lean protein diet will be surprisingly filling and satisfying.

Phase 1 of the Omni Diet is all about preparing for, and then making the leap. It has six steps. Start on all of them during your first week. Next week we'll add refinements and personalize the diet for you. But for now, Jump the Canyon!

- **Step 1: Know Your Numbers** – If possible, pay a visit to your doctor and get yourself measured on all the important numbers we just looked at.

- **Step 2: Purge Your Pantry** – Be ruthless. Get rid of all the food in your cabinets, refrigerator, freezer, and hidden in your desk drawer, that are not part of your new healthy lifestyle.

- **Step 3: Stock Up on Staples** – Go to the grocery store with a new attitude. Use the shopping list in The Omni Diet or a more extensive version found in my free newsletter, "Tana's Pantry," at www.tanaamen.com. Discover new treasures in the produce, fish, and organic meat departments. And stay away from the highly processed food. Read labels. Be daring in your choices.

- **Step 4: Start Moving Your Body** – Exercise is essential to your physical health and mental well-being. Surely you can fit in a 30-minute walk. Start there and your body will start craving exercise.

- **Step 5: Calculate Your Calorie Goals–Or Not!** – If you stick with the rules of the Omni Diet you will most likely see a sharp reduction in your calorie intake – even while you're eating more quantities of food. However, if you like to count calories, use the handy calorie counter on the Amen Clinics' Web site at www.amenclinics.com/cybcyb .

- **Step 6: Plan Your Meals** – Start by planning a few days ahead. As you get more familiar with the kind of food you're now eating, and you try out some of my recipes, it will be easier to do this. Use my two-week menu plans as a guide, but find foods that you like and that fit into your lifestyle. Rather than tracking meals as you go, use this Journal to plan meals by the week, or at least the night before. Then check off meals as you eat them.

[Discover a New World of Food]

EXERCISE

I'm all about "Replace, Don't Erase"! Great health is about abundance, not deprivation! When you jump the canyon it means giving up some foods that may have been favorites all your life. But you will likely be surprised to discover the amazing array of delicious, nutritious food you GET to eat on the Omni Diet.

Here's an exercise to follow this week that will get you started on your new food adventure!

- Look through my sample menu for this week and pick out a number of new items that seem interesting. Pick some breakfast smoothies, some lunch salads, and some dinner items. Use the planner to plan several days of menus in advance, rather than journaling your meals as you go. This will help to minimize impulsive decisions.

- Find instructions for preparing each dish in the recipe section of The Omni Diet. Prepare a shopping list of the ingredients you need to buy. To make it easy, use the electronic checklist found on the grocery list in "Tana's Pantry," my free newsletter. Go to www.tanaamen.com to get your free newsletter with weekly recipes, tips, and shopping list.

- If you fail to plan, you plan to fail! For best success, take a few hours each week to do your shopping, cut up veggies, boil a dozen eggs, bake a few chicken breasts or other favorite protein, and restock snack shelves. Measure out nuts and seeds into snack containers and make salad dressing.

- Go to the grocery store and buy what you need. While you're there investigate the other possibilities you may have never thought about before. Spend time in the produce department. If you're unsure about some of the fruits and vegetables, ask the produce manager about them. Most of the time they're delighted that someone is interested and will give you all kinds of valuable information. Pick up a few additional items that were not on your list, but that you'd now like to try.

- The next day, prepare and try your new foods. Eat mindfully. Savor each bite. Keep an open mind. And make notes of what you liked and how you could make it appeal to you more.

- A few days later, after you've tried everything, it's time to start over, planning, shopping, and preparing your meals. Make it a nutritional adventure and try new foods, or figure out what you like and stick with it. Either way, find your groove and plan ahead.

THE OMNI DIET DAILY JOURNAL
PHASE ONE-WEEK ONE

THE OMNI DIET DAILY JOURNAL

If You Fail to Plan, You Plan to Fail. Plan Your Meals for Tomorrow.

DAY ONE	Date _____		
Time	Food & Beverages	Calories	Healthy?
	Breakfast		Yes/No
	Snack		Yes/No
	Lunch		Yes/No
	Snack		Yes/No
	Dinner		Yes/No
	Other		Yes/No
	Total Calories Consumed		
	Total Liquid Calories Consumed		
	Total Calories Allowed		

THE OMNI DIET DAILY JOURNAL

Become A Warrior For Your Health! Phase One-Week One

DAY ONE

What is my desired outcome for the day? (Why MUST I do this?)

_____

_____

Three Things I am Grateful for Today:

1. _____

2. _____

3. _____

Today's Weight	Hours Slept Last Night	Managed stress ?

On a scale of 1 to 10 rate the following: (1 = poor, 10 = great)			
Mood	Energy	Digestion	Other Symptoms

Write your own mantra. Say it until you believe it.

_____

_____

Choose 5 healthy habits from the list below.

☐ Exercise 1 extra day each week ☐ Drink fresh green drinks 2X a week

☐ Lift weights at least 2X each week ☐ Go in the sauna 2X each week

☐ Drink 1 extra glass of water daily ☐ Write 5 things you're grateful for each morning

☐ Eat 1 extra cup of vegetables daily ☐ Mentor someone who wants improved health

☐ Write in a food journal every day ☐ List your daily victories in a victory journal

☐ Find an accountability buddy (AB) ☐ Review your goals and values

☐ Talk to your AB 2X each week ☐ Pray/meditate for 5 minutes daily

☐ Do "The Work of Byron Katie": www.thework.com

☐ Post a photo of someone you admire who mirrors your goals

MOTIVATIONAL BLAST:

The most dangerous thing in the world is to try to leap a chasm in two jumps.
— David Lloyd George

THE OMNI DIET DAILY JOURNAL

If You Fail to Plan, You Plan to Fail. Plan Your Meals for Tomorrow.

Time	DAY TWO	Food & Beverages	Date _____	Calories	Healthy?
	Breakfast				Yes/No
	Snack				Yes/No
	Lunch				Yes/No
	Snack				Yes/No
	Dinner				Yes/No
	Other				Yes/No
	Total Calories Consumed				
	Total Liquid Calories Consumed				
	Total Calories Allowed				

THE OMNI DIET DAILY JOURNAL
Become A Warrior For Your Health! Phase One-Week One

DAY TWO

What is my desired outcome for the day? (Why MUST I do this?)

_____

_____

Three Things I am Grateful for Today:

1. _____

2. _____

3. _____

Today's Weight	Hours Slept Last Night	Managed stress ?

On a scale of 1 to 10 rate the following: (1 = poor, 10 = great)			
Mood	Energy	Digestion	Other Symptoms

Write your own mantra. Say it until you believe it.

_____

_____

Choose 5 healthy habits from the list below.

☐ Exercise 1 extra day each week   ☐ Drink fresh green drinks 2X a week

☐ Lift weights at least 2X each week   ☐ Go in the sauna 2X each week

☐ Drink 1 extra glass of water daily   ☐ Write 5 things you're grateful for each morning

☐ Eat 1 extra cup of vegetables daily   ☐ Mentor someone who wants improved health

☐ Write in a food journal every day   ☐ List your daily victories in a victory journal

☐ Find an accountability buddy (AB)   ☐ Review your goals and values

☐ Talk to your AB 2X each week   ☐ Pray/meditate for 5 minutes daily

☐ Do "The Work of Byron Katie": www.thework.com

☐ Post a photo of someone you admire who mirrors your goals

MOTIVATIONAL BLAST:

On each side of the river grew a tree of life, bearing twelve crops of fruit, with a fresh crop each month. The leaves were used for medicine to heal the nations. — Holy Bible

THE OMNI DIET DAILY JOURNAL

If You Fail to Plan, You Plan to Fail. Plan Your Meals for Tomorrow.

| | DAY THREE | Date _____ | | |
Time	Food & Beverages		Calories	Healthy?
	Breakfast			Yes/No
	Snack			Yes/No
	Lunch			Yes/No
	Snack			Yes/No
	Dinner			Yes/No
	Other			Yes/No
	Total Calories Consumed			
	Total Liquid Calories Consumed			
	Total Calories Allowed			

THE OMNI DIET DAILY JOURNAL

Become A Warrior For Your Health! Phase One-Week One

What is my desired outcome for the day? (Why MUST I do this?)

_____

_____

Three Things I am Grateful for Today:

1. _____

2. _____

3. _____

Today's Weight	Hours Slept Last Night	Managed stress ?

On a scale of 1 to 10 rate the following: (1 = poor, 10 = great)			
Mood	Energy	Digestion	Other Symptoms

Write your own mantra. Say it until you believe it.

_____

_____

Choose 5 healthy habits from the list below.

- ☐ Exercise 1 extra day each week
- ☐ Lift weights at least 2X each week
- ☐ Drink 1 extra glass of water daily
- ☐ Eat 1 extra cup of vegetables daily
- ☐ Write in a food journal every day
- ☐ Find an accountability buddy (AB)
- ☐ Talk to your AB 2X each week
- ☐ Drink fresh green drinks 2X a week
- ☐ Go in the sauna 2X each week
- ☐ Write 5 things you're grateful for each morning
- ☐ Mentor someone who wants improved health
- ☐ List your daily victories in a victory journal
- ☐ Review your goals and values
- ☐ Pray/meditate for 5 minutes daily
- ☐ Do "The Work of Byron Katie": www.thework.com
- ☐ Post a photo of someone you admire who mirrors your goals

MOTIVATIONAL BLAST:

The greatest wealth is health. — Virgil

THE OMNI DIET DAILY JOURNAL

If You Fail to Plan, You Plan to Fail. Plan Your Meals for Tomorrow.

DAY FOUR		Date _____	
Time	**Food & Beverages**	**Calories**	**Healthy?**
Breakfast			Yes/No
Snack			Yes/No
Lunch			Yes/No
Snack			Yes/No
Dinner			Yes/No
Other			Yes/No
	Total Calories Consumed		
	Total Liquid Calories Consumed		
	Total Calories Allowed		

THE OMNI DIET DAILY JOURNAL

Become A Warrior For Your Health! Phase One-Week One

What is my desired outcome for the day? (Why MUST I do this?)

_____

_____

Three Things I am Grateful for Today:

1. _____

2. _____

3. _____

Today's Weight	Hours Slept Last Night	Managed stress ?

On a scale of 1 to 10 rate the following: (1 = poor, 10 = great)			
Mood	Energy	Digestion	Other Symptoms

Write your own mantra. Say it until you believe it.

_____

_____

Choose 5 healthy habits from the list below.

☐ Exercise 1 extra day each week   ☐ Drink fresh green drinks 2X a week

☐ Lift weights at least 2X each week   ☐ Go in the sauna 2X each week

☐ Drink 1 extra glass of water daily   ☐ Write 5 things you're grateful for each morning

☐ Eat 1 extra cup of vegetables daily   ☐ Mentor someone who wants improved health

☐ Write in a food journal every day   ☐ List your daily victories in a victory journal

☐ Find an accountability buddy (AB)   ☐ Review your goals and values

☐ Talk to your AB 2X each week   ☐ Pray/meditate for 5 minutes daily

☐ Do "The Work of Byron Katie": www.thework.com

☐ Post a photo of someone you admire who mirrors your goals

MOTIVATIONAL BLAST:

A healthy attitude is contagious but don't wait to catch it from others. Be a carrier.
— Tom Stoppard

THE OMNI DIET DAILY JOURNAL

If You Fail to Plan, You Plan to Fail. Plan Your Meals for Tomorrow.

	DAY FIVE	Date _____	
Time	**Food & Beverages**	**Calories**	**Healthy?**
	Breakfast		Yes/No
	Snack		Yes/No
	Lunch		Yes/No
	Snack		Yes/No
	Dinner		Yes/No
	Other		Yes/No
	Total Calories Consumed		
	Total Liquid Calories Consumed		
	Total Calories Allowed		

THE OMNI DIET DAILY JOURNAL

Become A Warrior For Your Health! Phase One-Week One

DAY FIVE

What is my desired outcome for the day? (Why MUST I do this?)

_____

_____

Three Things I am Grateful for Today:

1. _____

2. _____

3. _____

Today's Weight	Hours Slept Last Night	Managed stress ?

On a scale of 1 to 10 rate the following: (1 = poor, 10 = great)			
Mood	Energy	Digestion	Other Symptoms

Write your own mantra. Say it until you believe it.

_____

_____

Choose 5 healthy habits from the list below.

☐ Exercise 1 extra day each week   ☐ Drink fresh green drinks 2X a week

☐ Lift weights at least 2X each week   ☐ Go in the sauna 2X each week

☐ Drink 1 extra glass of water daily   ☐ Write 5 things you're grateful for each morning

☐ Eat 1 extra cup of vegetables daily   ☐ Mentor someone who wants improved health

☐ Write in a food journal every day   ☐ List your daily victories in a victory journal

☐ Find an accountability buddy (AB)   ☐ Review your goals and values

☐ Talk to your AB 2X each week   ☐ Pray/meditate for 5 minutes daily

☐ Do "The Work of Byron Katie": www.thework.com

☐ Post a photo of someone you admire who mirrors your goals

MOTIVATIONAL BLAST:

He who has health, has hope. And he who has hope, has everything. — _Arabian Proverb_

THE OMNI DIET DAILY JOURNAL

If You Fail to Plan, You Plan to Fail. Plan Your Meals for Tomorrow.

Time	DAY SIX — Food & Beverages	Date _____ Calories	Healthy?
	Breakfast		Yes/No
	Snack		Yes/No
	Lunch		Yes/No
	Snack		Yes/No
	Dinner		Yes/No
	Other		Yes/No
	Total Calories Consumed		
	Total Liquid Calories Consumed		
	Total Calories Allowed		

THE OMNI DIET DAILY JOURNAL
Become A Warrior For Your Health! Phase One-Week One

What is my desired outcome for the day? (Why MUST I do this?)

_____

_____

Three Things I am Grateful for Today:

1. _____

2. _____

3. _____

Today's Weight	Hours Slept Last Night	Managed stress ?

On a scale of 1 to 10 rate the following: (1 = poor, 10 = great)			
Mood	Energy	Digestion	Other Symptoms

Write your own mantra. Say it until you believe it.

_____

_____

Choose 5 healthy habits from the list below.

☐ Exercise 1 extra day each week   ☐ Drink fresh green drinks 2X a week

☐ Lift weights at least 2X each week   ☐ Go in the sauna 2X each week

☐ Drink 1 extra glass of water daily   ☐ Write 5 things you're grateful for each morning

☐ Eat 1 extra cup of vegetables daily   ☐ Mentor someone who wants improved health

☐ Write in a food journal every day   ☐ List your daily victories in a victory journal

☐ Find an accountability buddy (AB)   ☐ Review your goals and values

☐ Talk to your AB 2X each week   ☐ Pray/meditate for 5 minutes daily

☐ Do "The Work of Byron Katie": www.thework.com

☐ Post a photo of someone you admire who mirrors your goals

MOTIVATIONAL BLAST:

You can set yourself up to be sick, or you can choose to stay well. — Wayne Dyer

THE OMNI DIET DAILY JOURNAL

If You Fail to Plan, You Plan to Fail. Plan Your Meals for Tomorrow.

	DAY SEVEN	Date _____	
Time	**Food & Beverages**	**Calories**	**Healthy?**
	Breakfast		Yes/No
	Snack		Yes/No
	Lunch		Yes/No
	Snack		Yes/No
	Dinner		Yes/No
	Other		Yes/No
	Total Calories Consumed		
	Total Liquid Calories Consumed		
	Total Calories Allowed		

THE OMNI DIET DAILY JOURNAL

Become A Warrior For Your Health! Phase One-Week One

DAY SEVEN

What is my desired outcome for the day? (Why MUST I do this?)

_____

_____

Three Things I am Grateful for Today:

1. _____

2. _____

3. _____

Today's Weight	Hours Slept Last Night	Managed stress ?

On a scale of 1 to 10 rate the following: (1 = poor, 10 = great)			
Mood	Energy	Digestion	Other Symptoms

Write your own mantra. Say it until you believe it.

_____

_____

Choose 5 healthy habits from the list below.

☐ Exercise 1 extra day each week   ☐ Drink fresh green drinks 2X a week

☐ Lift weights at least 2X each week   ☐ Go in the sauna 2X each week

☐ Drink 1 extra glass of water daily   ☐ Write 5 things you're grateful for each morning

☐ Eat 1 extra cup of vegetables daily   ☐ Mentor someone who wants improved health

☐ Write in a food journal every day   ☐ List your daily victories in a victory journal

☐ Find an accountability buddy (AB)   ☐ Review your goals and values

☐ Talk to your AB 2X each week   ☐ Pray/meditate for 5 minutes daily

☐ Do "The Work of Byron Katie": www.thework.com

☐ Post a photo of someone you admire who mirrors your goals

MOTIVATIONAL BLAST:

It is only the first step that is difficult. — Marie De Vichy-Chamrond

THE OMNI DIET DAILY JOURNAL
PHASE ONE-WEEK ONE SUMMARY

	This Week	*Goal for Next Week*
Weight		
Number of Days I Slept 7 or More Hours		
Number of Days I Exercised at Least 30 Minutes		
Number of Days I Drank My Water Requirement		
Number of Days I Stayed Under My Allowed Calories		
Overall Weekly Energy Level (Low/Average/Good)		

Did I Accomplish My Goals Set This Week? (Circle One)		
Achieved	Over Achieved	Will Try Again!

My struggles this week were:

_____

_____

_____

_____

Ways I can achieve my goals next week:

_____

_____

_____

_____

My biggest accomplishment this week:

_____

_____

_____

Jump The Canyon

HOW TO STAY ON THE OTHER SIDE

You've jumped to the other side of the canyon! Great! Now we want to make sure you stay there. That means tailoring the Omni Diet so it fits your particular tastes and lifestyle, and finding tricks and tools to help you when cravings hit or temptation beckons. Here are some places to get started:

- **What do you love?** You are more likely to succeed on The Omni Diet if you discover an amazing array of foods that satisfy you. It may take some experimenting, but find acceptable foods that you love, and build your meal plans around them.

- **Always have a snack planned and handy.** Snacks are an important part of the Omni Diet, especially in the beginning when you are breaking food addictions. You don't want to let yourself get too hungry. It could play havoc with your blood sugar, and the next thing you know you might find yourself at a drive-thru window. So, wherever you go, carry single-size portions of snacks you enjoy.

- **Create a pattern interrupt.** You may occasionally be hit by a craving when you least expect it, especially when surprised by the familiar aroma of mom's home cooked food. Don't be blindsided. Have a plan in place to refocus your attention: take a walk, call a friend, eat a healthy snack, drink water – whatever works for you. If nothing works, allow a small cheat. Eat three bites of the food, enjoy it, and then throw away the rest. Don't let a small cheat become an excuse to go on a mindless binge.

- **Have a plan before you enter a restaurant.** You're meeting friends for lunch, or your spouse for a romantic dinner. Check out the menu online before you get there. Don't be afraid to custom order off of the menu;

most restaurants are happy to accommodate your needs. Don't allow the waiter to leave bread on the table! If others want it to stay, don't pout. Ask for some fresh veggies and guacamole. Be an example. Remember, you are a WARRIOR for your health.

- **Head off your excuses.** "I'm too tired to cook tonight." "I don't have anything healthy to eat." Take a few hours, one day each week to shop, chop, grill, and prepare. And when you do cook, always make enough food so you have healthy extra meals all ready for you if you don't feel like cooking. Set yourself up for success!

- **Give yourself time.** If you're rushing to get out the door in the morning you will be in danger of skipping breakfast. Healthy eating requires time – time to prepare, and time to enjoy. If you aren't a morning person, prepare everything the night before. Or get up half an hour earlier and give yourself the time you need.

I hope you get the idea. Personalize the Omni Diet for YOU, and YOU will stick with it

Refine and Personalize Your Omni Diet

EXERCISE

Now, let's make a list of ways you can personalize the Omni Diet to make it work for you!

These are some healthy foods I love:

_____

_____

_____

_____

These are some of my favorite snacks that I can easily keep handy:

_____

_____

_____

_____

When cravings hit, here is how I can distract myself:

_____

_____

Here are some possible menu choices at my favorite restaurants:

_____

_____

_____

_____

These are my favorite forms of exercise:

_____

_____

_____

_____

Here are some ways I'll head off my excuses for not exercising or eating right:

_____

_____

_____

_____

This is how I'll give myself more time to exercise and to prepare and enjoy my meals.

_____

_____

_____

_____

THE OMNI DIET DAILY JOURNAL
PHASE ONE-WEEK TWO

THE OMNI DIET DAILY JOURNAL

If You Fail to Plan, You Plan to Fail. Plan Your Meals for Tomorrow.

	DAY ONE	Date		
Time	Food & Beverages		Calories	Healthy?
Breakfast				Yes/No
Snack				Yes/No
Lunch				Yes/No
Snack				Yes/No
Dinner				Yes/No
Other				Yes/No
	Total Calories Consumed			
	Total Liquid Calories Consumed			
	Total Calories Allowed			

THE OMNI DIET DAILY JOURNAL

Become A Warrior For Your Health! Phase One-Week Two

DAY ONE

What is my desired outcome for the day? (Why MUST I do this?)

_____

_____

Three Things I am Grateful for Today:

1. _____

2. _____

3. _____

Today's Weight	Hours Slept Last Night	Managed stress ?

On a scale of 1 to 10 rate the following: (1 = poor, 10 = great)			
Mood	Energy	Digestion	Other Symptoms

Write your own mantra. Say it until you believe it.

_____

_____

Choose 5 healthy habits from the list below.

☐ Exercise 1 extra day each week   ☐ Drink fresh green drinks 2X a week

☐ Lift weights at least 2X each week   ☐ Go in the sauna 2X each week

☐ Drink 1 extra glass of water daily   ☐ Write 5 things you're grateful for each morning

☐ Eat 1 extra cup of vegetables daily   ☐ Mentor someone who wants improved health

☐ Write in a food journal every day   ☐ List your daily victories in a victory journal

☐ Find an accountability buddy (AB)   ☐ Review your goals and values

☐ Talk to your AB 2X each week   ☐ Pray/meditate for 5 minutes daily

☐ Do "The Work of Byron Katie": www.thework.com

☐ Post a photo of someone you admire who mirrors your goals

MOTIVATIONAL BLAST:

It is never too late to be who you might have been. — George Eliot

THE OMNI DIET DAILY JOURNAL

If You Fail to Plan, You Plan to Fail. Plan Your Meals for Tomorrow.

| DAY TWO | Date _____ |

Time	Food & Beverages	Calories	Healthy?
	Breakfast		Yes/No
	Snack		Yes/No
	Lunch		Yes/No
	Snack		Yes/No
	Dinner		Yes/No
	Other		Yes/No
	Total Calories Consumed		
	Total Liquid Calories Consumed		
	Total Calories Allowed		

THE OMNI DIET DAILY JOURNAL

Become A Warrior For Your Health! Phase One-Week Two

DAY TWO

What is my desired outcome for the day? (Why MUST I do this?)

_____

_____

Three Things I am Grateful for Today:

1. _____

2. _____

3. _____

Today's Weight	Hours Slept Last Night	Managed stress ?

On a scale of 1 to 10 rate the following: (1 = poor, 10 = great)

Mood	Energy	Digestion	Other Symptoms

Write your own mantra. Say it until you believe it.

_____

_____

Choose 5 healthy habits from the list below.

- ☐ Exercise 1 extra day each week
- ☐ Lift weights at least 2X each week
- ☐ Drink 1 extra glass of water daily
- ☐ Eat 1 extra cup of vegetables daily
- ☐ Write in a food journal every day
- ☐ Find an accountability buddy (AB)
- ☐ Talk to your AB 2X each week
- ☐ Drink fresh green drinks 2X a week
- ☐ Go in the sauna 2X each week
- ☐ Write 5 things you're grateful for each morning
- ☐ Mentor someone who wants improved health
- ☐ List your daily victories in a victory journal
- ☐ Review your goals and values
- ☐ Pray/meditate for 5 minutes daily
- ☐ Do "The Work of Byron Katie": www.thework.com
- ☐ Post a photo of someone you admire who mirrors your goals

MOTIVATIONAL BLAST:

The groundwork of all happiness is health. — James Leigh Hunt

THE OMNI DIET DAILY JOURNAL

If You Fail to Plan, You Plan to Fail. Plan Your Meals for Tomorrow.

Time	DAY THREE	Date		

Time	Food & Beverages	Calories	Healthy?
	Breakfast		Yes/No
	Snack		Yes/No
	Lunch		Yes/No
	Snack		Yes/No
	Dinner		Yes/No
	Other		Yes/No
	Total Calories Consumed		
	Total Liquid Calories Consumed		
	Total Calories Allowed		

THE OMNI DIET DAILY JOURNAL

Become A Warrior For Your Health! Phase One-Week Two

DAY THREE

What is my desired outcome for the day? (Why MUST I do this?)

_____

_____

Three Things I am Grateful for Today:

1. _____

2. _____

3. _____

Today's Weight	Hours Slept Last Night	Managed stress ?

On a scale of 1 to 10 rate the following: (1 = poor, 10 = great)			
Mood	Energy	Digestion	Other Symptoms

Write your own mantra. Say it until you believe it.

_____

_____

Choose 5 healthy habits from the list below.

☐ Exercise 1 extra day each week   ☐ Drink fresh green drinks 2X a week

☐ Lift weights at least 2X each week   ☐ Go in the sauna 2X each week

☐ Drink 1 extra glass of water daily   ☐ Write 5 things you're grateful for each morning

☐ Eat 1 extra cup of vegetables daily   ☐ Mentor someone who wants improved health

☐ Write in a food journal every day   ☐ List your daily victories in a victory journal

☐ Find an accountability buddy (AB)   ☐ Review your goals and values

☐ Talk to your AB 2X each week   ☐ Pray/meditate for 5 minutes daily

☐ Do "The Work of Byron Katie": www.thework.com

☐ Post a photo of someone you admire who mirrors your goals

MOTIVATIONAL BLAST:

You must begin to think of yourself as becoming the person you want to be.
— David Viscott

THE OMNI DIET DAILY JOURNAL

If You Fail to Plan, You Plan to Fail. Plan Your Meals for Tomorrow.

Time	Food & Beverages	Calories	Healthy?
DAY FOUR	Date _____		
	Breakfast		Yes/No
	Snack		Yes/No
	Lunch		Yes/No
	Snack		Yes/No
	Dinner		Yes/No
	Other		Yes/No
	Total Calories Consumed		
	Total Liquid Calories Consumed		
	Total Calories Allowed		

THE OMNI DIET DAILY JOURNAL

Become A Warrior For Your Health! Phase One-Week Two

What is my desired outcome for the day? (Why MUST I do this?)

_____

_____

Three Things I am Grateful for Today:

1. _____

2. _____

3. _____

Today's Weight	Hours Slept Last Night	Managed stress ?

On a scale of 1 to 10 rate the following: (1 = poor, 10 = great)			
Mood	Energy	Digestion	Other Symptoms

Write your own mantra. Say it until you believe it.

_____

_____

Choose 5 healthy habits from the list below.

☐ Exercise 1 extra day each week   ☐ Drink fresh green drinks 2X a week

☐ Lift weights at least 2X each week   ☐ Go in the sauna 2X each week

☐ Drink 1 extra glass of water daily   ☐ Write 5 things you're grateful for each morning

☐ Eat 1 extra cup of vegetables daily   ☐ Mentor someone who wants improved health

☐ Write in a food journal every day   ☐ List your daily victories in a victory journal

☐ Find an accountability buddy (AB)   ☐ Review your goals and values

☐ Talk to your AB 2X each week   ☐ Pray/meditate for 5 minutes daily

☐ Do "The Work of Byron Katie": www.thework.com

☐ Post a photo of someone you admire who mirrors your goals

MOTIVATIONAL BLAST:

Though no one can go back and make a brand new start, anyone can start from now and make a brand new ending. — Carl Bard

THE OMNI DIET DAILY JOURNAL

If You Fail to Plan, You Plan to Fail. Plan Your Meals for Tomorrow.

Time	DAY FIVE — Food & Beverages	Date _____ Calories	Healthy?
Breakfast			Yes/No
Snack			Yes/No
Lunch			Yes/No
Snack			Yes/No
Dinner			Yes/No
Other			Yes/No
	Total Calories Consumed		
	Total Liquid Calories Consumed		
	Total Calories Allowed		

THE OMNI DIET DAILY JOURNAL

Become A Warrior For Your Health! Phase One-Week Two

What is my desired outcome for the day? (Why MUST I do this?)

_____

_____

Three Things I am Grateful for Today:

1. _____

2. _____

3. _____

Today's Weight	Hours Slept Last Night	Managed stress ?

On a scale of 1 to 10 rate the following: (1 = poor, 10 = great)			
Mood	Energy	Digestion	Other Symptoms

Write your own mantra. Say it until you believe it.

_____

_____

Choose 5 healthy habits from the list below.

- ☐ Exercise 1 extra day each week
- ☐ Lift weights at least 2X each week
- ☐ Drink 1 extra glass of water daily
- ☐ Eat 1 extra cup of vegetables daily
- ☐ Write in a food journal every day
- ☐ Find an accountability buddy (AB)
- ☐ Talk to your AB 2X each week
- ☐ Drink fresh green drinks 2X a week
- ☐ Go in the sauna 2X each week
- ☐ Write 5 things you're grateful for each morning
- ☐ Mentor someone who wants improved health
- ☐ List your daily victories in a victory journal
- ☐ Review your goals and values
- ☐ Pray/meditate for 5 minutes daily
- ☐ Do "The Work of Byron Katie": www.thework.com
- ☐ Post a photo of someone you admire who mirrors your goals

MOTIVATIONAL BLAST:

Take care of your body. It's the only place you have to live. — Jim Rohn

THE OMNI DIET DAILY JOURNAL
If You Fail to Plan, You Plan to Fail. Plan Your Meals for Tomorrow.

Time	DAY SIX	Date _____		
	Food & Beverages	**Calories**	**Healthy?**
	Breakfast		Yes/No
	Snack		Yes/No
	Lunch		Yes/No
	Snack		Yes/No
	Dinner		Yes/No
	Other		Yes/No
	Total Calories Consumed		
	Total Liquid Calories Consumed		
	Total Calories Allowed		

THE OMNI DIET DAILY JOURNAL

Become A Warrior For Your Health! Phase One-Week Two

DAY SIX

What is my desired outcome for the day? (Why MUST I do this?)

_____

_____

Three Things I am Grateful for Today:

1. _____

2. _____

3. _____

Today's Weight	Hours Slept Last Night	Managed stress ?

On a scale of 1 to 10 rate the following: (1 = poor, 10 = great)			
Mood	Energy	Digestion	Other Symptoms

Write your own mantra. Say it until you believe it.

_____

_____

Choose 5 healthy habits from the list below.

☐ Exercise 1 extra day each week

☐ Lift weights at least 2X each week

☐ Drink 1 extra glass of water daily

☐ Eat 1 extra cup of vegetables daily

☐ Write in a food journal every day

☐ Find an accountability buddy (AB)

☐ Talk to your AB 2X each week

☐ Drink fresh green drinks 2X a week

☐ Go in the sauna 2X each week

☐ Write 5 things you're grateful for each morning

☐ Mentor someone who wants improved health

☐ List your daily victories in a victory journal

☐ Review your goals and values

☐ Pray/meditate for 5 minutes daily

☐ Do "The Work of Byron Katie": www.thework.com

☐ Post a photo of someone you admire who mirrors your goals

MOTIVATIONAL BLAST:

Taking joy in living is a woman's best cosmetic. — Rosalind Russell

THE OMNI DIET DAILY JOURNAL

If You Fail to Plan, You Plan to Fail. Plan Your Meals for Tomorrow.

DAY SEVEN	Date

Time	Food & Beverages	Calories	Healthy?
Breakfast			Yes/No
Snack			Yes/No
Lunch			Yes/No
Snack			Yes/No
Dinner			Yes/No
Other			Yes/No
	Total Calories Consumed	
	Total Liquid Calories Consumed	
	Total Calories Allowed	

THE OMNI DIET DAILY JOURNAL

Become A Warrior For Your Health! Phase One-Week Two

DAY SEVEN

What is my desired outcome for the day? (Why MUST I do this?)

_____

_____

Three Things I am Grateful for Today:

1. _____

2. _____

3. _____

Today's Weight	Hours Slept Last Night	Managed stress ?

On a scale of 1 to 10 rate the following: (1 = poor, 10 = great)			
Mood	Energy	Digestion	Other Symptoms

Write your own mantra. Say it until you believe it.

_____

_____

Choose 5 healthy habits from the list below.

☐ Exercise 1 extra day each week   ☐ Drink fresh green drinks 2X a week

☐ Lift weights at least 2X each week   ☐ Go in the sauna 2X each week

☐ Drink 1 extra glass of water daily   ☐ Write 5 things you're grateful for each morning

☐ Eat 1 extra cup of vegetables daily   ☐ Mentor someone who wants improved health

☐ Write in a food journal every day   ☐ List your daily victories in a victory journal

☐ Find an accountability buddy (AB)   ☐ Review your goals and values

☐ Talk to your AB 2X each week   ☐ Pray/meditate for 5 minutes daily

☐ Do "The Work of Byron Katie": www.thework.com

☐ Post a photo of someone you admire who mirrors your goals

MOTIVATIONAL BLAST:

Our bodies are our gardens – our wills are our gardeners. — William Shakespeare

THE OMNI DIET DAILY JOURNAL
PHASE ONE-WEEK TWO SUMMARY

	This Week	*Goal for Next Week*
Weight		
Number of Days I Slept 7 or More Hours		
Number of Days I Exercised at Least 30 Minutes		
Number of Days I Drank My Water Requirement		
Number of Days I Stayed Under My Allowed Calories		
Overall Weekly Energy Level (Low/Average/Good)		

Did I Accomplish My Goals Set This Week? (Circle One)		
Achieved	Over Achieved	Will Try Again!

My struggles this week were:

_____

_____

_____

_____

Ways I can achieve my goals next week:

_____

_____

_____

_____

My biggest accomplishment this week:

_____

_____

_____

[Pump It Up:]

STAY ON TRACK WITH A FOOD JOURNAL

During this phase of the Omni Diet, we want to ramp up every aspect of your program. But in my experience, when it comes to the diet part, this is when people may begin to relax on portion sizes or forget key rules and fall back into old habits.

One of the best antidotes I know is to become extremely conscious of everything you put in your mouth by writing it down in a food journal. It's a great way to understand your eating patterns—and an incredibly effective tool for Omni Diet success. Research shows (as does nearly every successful long-term program) that keeping a food journal is a critical tool for changing eating behavior.

Advantages of Keeping a Food Journal

- Provides hard evidence that you haven't been measuring your portion sizes correctly or you're not sticking to a proper meal schedule.

- Reveals how many calories you take in unconsciously with little bites and nibbles here and there that sabotage your success.

- Forces you to be completely aware of (and accountable for) the food choices you make.

- It's the best treatment I know for "food amnesia"—forgetting when you eat a few bites of your child's breakfast or polishing off the dinner leftovers that were supposed to be the next day's lunch, which can add hundreds of calories to your diet each day.

- Any format works— if you forget your journal, use a notebook, your phone, even a piece of paper taped to the refrigerator.

- Keep it simple: Whenever you eat something, write down the time, the food, and the portion size.

- Jot down other relevant notes, such as what events or situations preceded the meal or snack, whether you were stressed or had PMS, whether you were eating in response to a craving, etc. Just a few words are usually enough. It doesn't take much time at all.

- After a week of keeping a food journal, go through it and see what you notice. Usually, strong patterns pointing to unhealthy eating jump right out at you. For example, you may see that you make poor snack choices in the evening while you're watching TV. Or you may notice that hunger at 3 p.m. sends you off to the vending machines at work.

- Once you know and understand your negative eating patterns, you can devise solutions. If you like to eat in the evening, rearrange your meals to make room for an extra evening meal or snack. If you're very hungry at 3 p.m., shift some of your dinner calories to mid-afternoon and keep healthy snacks close at hand. Once you know your weak points, you can address them in a healthy way.

Don't worry—you don't have to keep this up forever (but many do because it helps them so much). Keeping a food journal for the first three phases gives you valuable information about your eating habits.

Start Your Food Journal

EXERCISE

You've already got a great start to a food journal. It's the list of foods you plan each day for the next day, and that you check off as you eat each meal. You just need to keep a record of some additional information. Here are some ideas for the kind of record you can keep.

List any snacks, nibbles, or tastes that you ate in addition to your planned meals for the day. Write down the time it was when you ate, what you ate, the quantity, and a description of the situation that led to eating. This will help you see if there are any patterns you need to break. Your record can look like this:

Time	What I ate	Amount I ate	Event or Situation prior to snacking

Were you responding to cravings? By seeing a pattern in your cravings you can begin to plan to "head them off" rather than caving in to them. Describe any cravings here, write down the time you had them, and describe how you responded to them:

_____

_____

_____

_____

Write down how you felt this day, again to see if there are any patterns. Were you anxious and stressed? Depressed? Happy and carefree? Did you have PMS? Did you have menopausal symptoms?

_____

_____

_____

_____

At the end of each week, review your food journal to see what patterns emerge, and how you're changing as you stick with the Omni Diet.

THE OMNI DIET DAILY JOURNAL
PHASE TWO-WEEK ONE

THE OMNI DIET DAILY JOURNAL

If You Fail to Plan, You Plan to Fail. Plan Your Meals for Tomorrow.

	DAY ONE		Date	
Time	**Food & Beverages**		**Calories**	**Healthy?**
	Breakfast			Yes/No
	Snack			Yes/No
	Lunch			Yes/No
	Snack			Yes/No
	Dinner			Yes/No
	Other			Yes/No
	Total Calories Consumed			
	Total Liquid Calories Consumed			
	Total Calories Allowed			

THE OMNI DIET DAILY JOURNAL
Become A Warrior For Your Health! Phase Two-Week One

What is my desired outcome for the day? (Why MUST I do this?)

_____

_____

Three Things I am Grateful for Today:

1. _____

2. _____

3. _____

Today's Weight	Hours Slept Last Night	Managed stress ?

On a scale of 1 to 10 rate the following: (1 = poor, 10 = great)			
Mood	Energy	Digestion	Other Symptoms

Write your own mantra. Say it until you believe it.

_____

_____

Choose 5 healthy habits from the list below.

☐ Exercise 1 extra day each week

☐ Lift weights at least 2X each week

☐ Drink 1 extra glass of water daily

☐ Eat 1 extra cup of vegetables daily

☐ Write in a food journal every day

☐ Find an accountability buddy (AB)

☐ Talk to your AB 2X each week

☐ Drink fresh green drinks 2X a week

☐ Go in the sauna 2X each week

☐ Write 5 things you're grateful for each morning

☐ Mentor someone who wants improved health

☐ List your daily victories in a victory journal

☐ Review your goals and values

☐ Pray/meditate for 5 minutes daily

☐ Do "The Work of Byron Katie": www.thework.com

☐ Post a photo of someone you admire who mirrors your goals

MOTIVATIONAL BLAST:

To eat is a necessity, but to eat intelligently is an art. — La Rochefoucauld

THE OMNI DIET DAILY JOURNAL

If You Fail to Plan, You Plan to Fail. Plan Your Meals for Tomorrow.

	DAY TWO	Date _____		
Time	Food & Beverages		Calories	Healthy?
Breakfast				Yes/No
Snack				Yes/No
Lunch				Yes/No
Snack				Yes/No
Dinner				Yes/No
Other				Yes/No
	Total Calories Consumed			
	Total Liquid Calories Consumed			
	Total Calories Allowed			

THE OMNI DIET DAILY JOURNAL

Become A Warrior For Your Health! Phase Two-Week One

What is my desired outcome for the day? (Why MUST I do this?)

_____

_____

Three Things I am Grateful for Today:

1. _____

2. _____

3. _____

Today's Weight	Hours Slept Last Night	Managed stress ?

On a scale of 1 to 10 rate the following: (1 = poor, 10 = great)			
Mood	Energy	Digestion	Other Symptoms

Write your own mantra. Say it until you believe it.

_____

_____

Choose 5 healthy habits from the list below.

☐ Exercise 1 extra day each week ☐ Drink fresh green drinks 2X a week

☐ Lift weights at least 2X each week ☐ Go in the sauna 2X each week

☐ Drink 1 extra glass of water daily ☐ Write 5 things you're grateful for each morning

☐ Eat 1 extra cup of vegetables daily ☐ Mentor someone who wants improved health

☐ Write in a food journal every day ☐ List your daily victories in a victory journal

☐ Find an accountability buddy (AB) ☐ Review your goals and values

☐ Talk to your AB 2X each week ☐ Pray/meditate for 5 minutes daily

☐ Do "The Work of Byron Katie": www.thework.com

☐ Post a photo of someone you admire who mirrors your goals

MOTIVATIONAL BLAST:

Motivation is what gets you started. Habit is what keeps you going. — Jim Ryun

THE OMNI DIET DAILY JOURNAL

If You Fail to Plan, You Plan to Fail. Plan Your Meals for Tomorrow.

	DAY THREE	Date _____	
Time	**Food & Beverages**	**Calories**	**Healthy?**
	Breakfast		Yes/No
	Snack		Yes/No
	Lunch		Yes/No
	Snack		Yes/No
	Dinner		Yes/No
	Other		Yes/No
	Total Calories Consumed		
	Total Liquid Calories Consumed		
	Total Calories Allowed		

THE OMNI DIET DAILY JOURNAL

Become A Warrior For Your Health! Phase Two-Week One

What is my desired outcome for the day? (Why MUST I do this?)

_____

_____

Three Things I am Grateful for Today:

1. _____

2. _____

3. _____

Today's Weight	Hours Slept Last Night	Managed stress ?

On a scale of 1 to 10 rate the following: (1 = poor, 10 = great)			
Mood	Energy	Digestion	Other Symptoms

Write your own mantra. Say it until you believe it.

_____

_____

Choose 5 healthy habits from the list below.

☐ Exercise 1 extra day each week   ☐ Drink fresh green drinks 2X a week

☐ Lift weights at least 2X each week   ☐ Go in the sauna 2X each week

☐ Drink 1 extra glass of water daily   ☐ Write 5 things you're grateful for each morning

☐ Eat 1 extra cup of vegetables daily   ☐ Mentor someone who wants improved health

☐ Write in a food journal every day   ☐ List your daily victories in a victory journal

☐ Find an accountability buddy (AB)   ☐ Review your goals and values

☐ Talk to your AB 2X each week   ☐ Pray/meditate for 5 minutes daily

☐ Do "The Work of Byron Katie": www.thework.com

☐ Post a photo of someone you admire who mirrors your goals

MOTIVATIONAL BLAST:

I know for sure that what we dwell on is who we become. — Oprah Winfrey

THE OMNI DIET DAILY JOURNAL

If You Fail to Plan, You Plan to Fail. Plan Your Meals for Tomorrow.

DAY FOUR		Date _____		
Time	Food & Beverages		Calories	Healthy?
Breakfast				Yes/No
Snack				Yes/No
Lunch				Yes/No
Snack				Yes/No
Dinner				Yes/No
Other				Yes/No
	Total Calories Consumed			
	Total Liquid Calories Consumed			
	Total Calories Allowed			

THE OMNI DIET DAILY JOURNAL

Become A Warrior For Your Health! Phase Two-Week One

DAY FOUR

What is my desired outcome for the day? (Why MUST I do this?)

_____

_____

Three Things I am Grateful for Today:

1. _____

2. _____

3. _____

Today's Weight	Hours Slept Last Night	Managed stress ?

On a scale of 1 to 10 rate the following: (1 = poor, 10 = great)			
Mood	Energy	Digestion	Other Symptoms

Write your own mantra. Say it until you believe it.

_____

_____

Choose 5 healthy habits from the list below.

☐ Exercise 1 extra day each week

☐ Lift weights at least 2X each week

☐ Drink 1 extra glass of water daily

☐ Eat 1 extra cup of vegetables daily

☐ Write in a food journal every day

☐ Find an accountability buddy (AB)

☐ Talk to your AB 2X each week

☐ Do "The Work of Byron Katie": www.thework.com

☐ Post a photo of someone you admire who mirrors your goals

☐ Drink fresh green drinks 2X a week

☐ Go in the sauna 2X each week

☐ Write 5 things you're grateful for each morning

☐ Mentor someone who wants improved health

☐ List your daily victories in a victory journal

☐ Review your goals and values

☐ Pray/meditate for 5 minutes daily

MOTIVATIONAL BLAST:

The wise man should consider that health is the greatest of human blessings. Let food be your medicine. — Hippocrates

THE OMNI DIET DAILY JOURNAL

If You Fail to Plan, You Plan to Fail. Plan Your Meals for Tomorrow.

| DAY FIVE | Date _____ | | |

Time	Food & Beverages	Calories	Healthy?
Breakfast			Yes/No
Snack			Yes/No
Lunch			Yes/No
Snack			Yes/No
Dinner			Yes/No
Other			Yes/No
	Total Calories Consumed		
	Total Liquid Calories Consumed		
	Total Calories Allowed		

THE OMNI DIET DAILY JOURNAL

Become A Warrior For Your Health! Phase Two-Week One

What is my desired outcome for the day? (Why MUST I do this?)

_____

_____

Three Things I am Grateful for Today:

1. _____

2. _____

3. _____

Today's Weight	Hours Slept Last Night	Managed stress ?

On a scale of 1 to 10 rate the following: (1 = poor, 10 = great)			
Mood	Energy	Digestion	Other Symptoms

Write your own mantra. Say it until you believe it.

_____

_____

Choose 5 healthy habits from the list below.

☐ Exercise 1 extra day each week
☐ Lift weights at least 2X each week
☐ Drink 1 extra glass of water daily
☐ Eat 1 extra cup of vegetables daily
☐ Write in a food journal every day
☐ Find an accountability buddy (AB)
☐ Talk to your AB 2X each week
☐ Do "The Work of Byron Katie": www.thework.com
☐ Post a photo of someone you admire who mirrors your goals

☐ Drink fresh green drinks 2X a week
☐ Go in the sauna 2X each week
☐ Write 5 things you're grateful for each morning
☐ Mentor someone who wants improved health
☐ List your daily victories in a victory journal
☐ Review your goals and values
☐ Pray/meditate for 5 minutes daily

MOTIVATIONAL BLAST:

To insure good health: eat lightly, breathe deeply, live moderately, cultivate cheerfulness, and maintain an interest in life. — William Londen

THE OMNI DIET DAILY JOURNAL

If You Fail to Plan, You Plan to Fail. Plan Your Meals for Tomorrow.

	DAY SIX	Date	
Time	**Food & Beverages**	**Calories**	**Healthy?**
	Breakfast		Yes/No
	Snack		Yes/No
	Lunch		Yes/No
	Snack		Yes/No
	Dinner		Yes/No
	Other		Yes/No
	Total Calories Consumed		
	Total Liquid Calories Consumed		
	Total Calories Allowed		

THE OMNI DIET DAILY JOURNAL

Become A Warrior For Your Health! Phase Two-Week One

DAY SIX

What is my desired outcome for the day? (Why MUST I do this?)

_____

_____

Three Things I am Grateful for Today:

1. _____

2. _____

3. _____

Today's Weight	Hours Slept Last Night	Managed stress ?

On a scale of 1 to 10 rate the following: (1 = poor, 10 = great)			
Mood	Energy	Digestion	Other Symptoms

Write your own mantra. Say it until you believe it.

_____

_____

Choose 5 healthy habits from the list below.

☐ Exercise 1 extra day each week   ☐ Drink fresh green drinks 2X a week

☐ Lift weights at least 2X each week   ☐ Go in the sauna 2X each week

☐ Drink 1 extra glass of water daily   ☐ Write 5 things you're grateful for each morning

☐ Eat 1 extra cup of vegetables daily   ☐ Mentor someone who wants improved health

☐ Write in a food journal every day   ☐ List your daily victories in a victory journal

☐ Find an accountability buddy (AB)   ☐ Review your goals and values

☐ Talk to your AB 2X each week   ☐ Pray/meditate for 5 minutes daily

☐ Do "The Work of Byron Katie": www.thework.com

☐ Post a photo of someone you admire who mirrors your goals

MOTIVATIONAL BLAST:

Did you ever stop to taste a carrot? Not just eat it, but taste it? You can't taste the beauty and energy of the earth in a Twinkie. — Astrid Alauda

THE OMNI DIET DAILY JOURNAL

If You Fail to Plan, You Plan to Fail. Plan Your Meals for Tomorrow.

Time	Food & Beverages	Calories	Healthy?
DAY SEVEN		Date	
Breakfast			Yes/No
Snack			Yes/No
Lunch			Yes/No
Snack			Yes/No
Dinner			Yes/No
Other			Yes/No
	Total Calories Consumed		
	Total Liquid Calories Consumed		
	Total Calories Allowed		

THE OMNI DIET DAILY JOURNAL

Become A Warrior For Your Health! Phase Two-Week One

What is my desired outcome for the day? (Why MUST I do this?)

_____

_____

Three Things I am Grateful for Today:

1. _____

2. _____

3. _____

Today's Weight	Hours Slept Last Night	Managed stress ?

On a scale of 1 to 10 rate the following: (1 = poor, 10 = great)			
Mood	Energy	Digestion	Other Symptoms

Write your own mantra. Say it until you believe it.

_____

_____

Choose 5 healthy habits from the list below.

☐ Exercise 1 extra day each week   ☐ Drink fresh green drinks 2X a week

☐ Lift weights at least 2X each week   ☐ Go in the sauna 2X each week

☐ Drink 1 extra glass of water daily   ☐ Write 5 things you're grateful for each morning

☐ Eat 1 extra cup of vegetables daily   ☐ Mentor someone who wants improved health

☐ Write in a food journal every day   ☐ List your daily victories in a victory journal

☐ Find an accountability buddy (AB)   ☐ Review your goals and values

☐ Talk to your AB 2X each week   ☐ Pray/meditate for 5 minutes daily

☐ Do "The Work of Byron Katie": www.thework.com

☐ Post a photo of someone you admire who mirrors your goals

MOTIVATIONAL BLAST:

Fall seven times, stand up eight. — Japanese Proverb

THE OMNI DIET DAILY JOURNAL
PHASE TWO - WEEK ONE SUMMARY

	This Week	*Goal for Next Week*
Weight		
Number of Days I Slept 7 or More Hours		
Number of Days I Exercised at Least 30 Minutes		
Number of Days I Drank My Water Requirement		
Number of Days I Stayed Under My Allowed Calories		
Overall Weekly Energy Level (Low/Average/Good)		

Did I Accomplish My Goals Set This Week? (Circle One)		
Achieved	Over Achieved	Will Try Again!

My struggles this week were:

_____

_____

_____

Ways I can achieve my goals next week:

_____

_____

_____

My biggest accomplishment this week:

_____

_____

_____

Pump It Up:

GET YOUR BODY MOVING

Regardless of your level of exercise prior to starting the Omni Diet, by now you should have at least started walking regularly. With two weeks of walking under your belt, you should now be ready for a more ambitious exercise regimen with two components: Interval Training and Strength Training.

The Omni Interval Training Workout

- Interval training alternates moderate exercise with bursts of intensity. You work at a moderate pace, go all out at a high intensity for a short period of time, and then return to your initial moderate pace. Repeat the cycle throughout your workout.

- For example, you may alternate three minutes of brisk walking with one minute of sprinting. Or on a bicycle, you may alternate several minutes of comfortable pedaling with a brief burst of intense pedaling. You can do interval training indoors on a treadmill, stationary cycle, or other cardiovascular gym machine, or outdoors while walking, jogging, or cycling.

- Let your fitness level determine your pace. Train for 20 to 30 minutes, but no longer. Begin with a moderate pace for 3 minutes, followed by a burst of maximum exertion for 30 seconds to 1 minute. Then repeat. Try to burst at least four times during an interval workout.

- If you are just starting to exercise and are overweight, your pace for interval training may be a slow walk. If you're already in good shape, you may be sprinting uphill. Either one is okay. Start where you are, and work up from there.

- If you're a beginner or if you have any medical conditions, I advise using a heart-rate (HR) monitor. You can get a decent one for about twenty-five dollars. Using an HR monitor helps you regulate your workouts and prevents you from exercising too intensely. Once you're in shape, you won't need it as much.

The Omni Strength Training Workout

- Instructions and diagrams for Omni Strength Training appear on pages 217-222 of The Omni Diet.

- I recommend doing the Omni Strength Training Workout three times a week, on Mondays, Wednesdays, and Fridays. Plan about 40 minutes per session. Other than comfortable clothes and sneakers, this workout requires little or no exercise equipment. If you can afford it, buy some dumbbells, also known as free weights. It's nice to have a workout bench, but if you don't, you can use a chair or bed. A HR monitor can be helpful.

- When you do your strength training exercises, be sure to rest between sets until your heart rate reaches about 60 percent of your maximum heart rate. This is your target heart rate. As you begin to increase your strength and endurance, you will naturally decrease the amount of rest time between sets.

- As your strength increases, get creative. If you don't have fancy gym equipment, run up a flight of stairs, add push ups and pull ups. Sprint uphill between sets of lifting weight.

Think like a WARRIOR! Act like a WARRIOR! Move like a WARRIOR!

Follow Your Exercise Program

EXERCISE

Start following the Omni Diet Workout, using the instructions on the previous page and in The Omni Diet.

This workout is the smartest way to exercise because it concentrates highly effective moves into a program that works your entire body. It combines interval training with weight training for maximum benefits in the shortest time. It can be done at home, in the gym, or even in a hotel room when you're on the road. You can adjust its intensity according to your current fitness level, and increase intensity as you become stronger. Before you get started, keep two things in mind:

- If you have a medical condition or if you've never engaged in regular exercise, be sure to get your doctor's approval before you start.

- Once you first start exercising, you may find that you feel so good that you overdo it. Try to hold back—the best, fastest way to achieve results is not to overtrain, but to train at optimal levels.

Your Workout Schedule for Best Results

- Mondays, Wednesdays, and Fridays: Strength train for about 40 minutes a day using the Omni Strength Training Workout.

- Tuesdays and Thursdays: Interval train for 30 minutes (20 minutes if you're a beginner) a day using the Omni Interval Training Workout.

- Saturdays: Interval train or take a leisurely 30-minute walk.

- Sundays: Rest and rejuvenate.

Your Heart's Best Beats

Exercise is most effective when the intensity level causes your heart to beat at specific rates, depending on the kind of exercise. To determine your optimal heart rates for various activities, follow these steps:

- For your maximum heart rate (MHR), subtract your age from 220. If you are fifty years old, for example, your maximum heart rate is 170.

- For your target heart rate (THR), multiply your MHR by 0.6 (60 percent) for strength training, 0.7 (70 percent) for cardiovascular training, and 0.85 (85 percent) for interval training.

- Check your HR monitor while you're working out. If your HR is too high, slow down a bit. If it's too low, push a little harder.

- Never let your heart rate exceed 85 percent of your MHR.

- If you have health problems, talk with your health-care provider about the right target heart rates for you.

THE OMNI DIET DAILY JOURNAL
PHASE TWO-WEEK TWO

THE OMNI DIET DAILY JOURNAL

If You Fail to Plan, You Plan to Fail. Plan Your Meals for Tomorrow.

| DAY ONE | Date _____ | | |

Time	Food & Beverages	Calories	Healthy?
Breakfast			Yes/No
Snack			Yes/No
Lunch			Yes/No
Snack			Yes/No
Dinner			Yes/No
Other			Yes/No
	Total Calories Consumed		
	Total Liquid Calories Consumed		
	Total Calories Allowed		

THE OMNI DIET DAILY JOURNAL

Become A Warrior For Your Health! Phase Two-Week Two

What is my desired outcome for the day? (Why MUST I do this?)

_____

_____

Three Things I am Grateful for Today:

1. _____

2. _____

3. _____

Today's Weight	Hours Slept Last Night	Managed stress ?

On a scale of 1 to 10 rate the following: (1 = poor, 10 = great)			
Mood	Energy	Digestion	Other Symptoms

Write your own mantra. Say it until you believe it.

_____

_____

Choose 5 healthy habits from the list below.

☐ Exercise 1 extra day each week   ☐ Drink fresh green drinks 2X a week

☐ Lift weights at least 2X each week   ☐ Go in the sauna 2X each week

☐ Drink 1 extra glass of water daily   ☐ Write 5 things you're grateful for each morning

☐ Eat 1 extra cup of vegetables daily   ☐ Mentor someone who wants improved health

☐ Write in a food journal every day   ☐ List your daily victories in a victory journal

☐ Find an accountability buddy (AB)   ☐ Review your goals and values

☐ Talk to your AB 2X each week   ☐ Pray/meditate for 5 minutes daily

☐ Do "The Work of Byron Katie": www.thework.com

☐ Post a photo of someone you admire who mirrors your goals

MOTIVATIONAL BLAST:

If we could give every individual the right amount of nourishment and exercise, not too little and not too much, we would have found the safest way to health. — Hippocrates

THE OMNI DIET DAILY JOURNAL

If You Fail to Plan, You Plan to Fail. Plan Your Meals for Tomorrow.

| | DAY TWO | Date _____ | | |
Time	Food & Beverages		Calories	Healthy?
	Breakfast			Yes/No
	Snack			Yes/No
	Lunch			Yes/No
	Snack			Yes/No
	Dinner			Yes/No
	Other			Yes/No
	Total Calories Consumed			
	Total Liquid Calories Consumed			
	Total Calories Allowed			

74

THE OMNI DIET DAILY JOURNAL

Become A Warrior For Your Health! Phase Two-Week Two

DAY TWO

What is my desired outcome for the day? (Why MUST I do this?)

_____

_____

Three Things I am Grateful for Today:

1. _____

2. _____

3. _____

Today's Weight	Hours Slept Last Night	Managed stress ?

On a scale of 1 to 10 rate the following: (1 = poor, 10 = great)			
Mood	Energy	Digestion	Other Symptoms

Write your own mantra. Say it until you believe it.

_____

_____

Choose 5 healthy habits from the list below.

☐ Exercise 1 extra day each week

☐ Lift weights at least 2X each week

☐ Drink 1 extra glass of water daily

☐ Eat 1 extra cup of vegetables daily

☐ Write in a food journal every day

☐ Find an accountability buddy (AB)

☐ Talk to your AB 2X each week

☐ Drink fresh green drinks 2X a week

☐ Go in the sauna 2X each week

☐ Write 5 things you're grateful for each morning

☐ Mentor someone who wants improved health

☐ List your daily victories in a victory journal

☐ Review your goals and values

☐ Pray/meditate for 5 minutes daily

☐ Do "The Work of Byron Katie": www.thework.com

☐ Post a photo of someone you admire who mirrors your goals

MOTIVATIONAL BLAST:

No matter how slow you go, you are still lapping everybody on the couch. — Unknown

THE OMNI DIET DAILY JOURNAL

If You Fail to Plan, You Plan to Fail. Plan Your Meals for Tomorrow.

	DAY THREE		Date	
Time	**Food & Beverages**	**Calories**	**Healthy?**	
Breakfast			Yes/No	
Snack			Yes/No	
Lunch			Yes/No	
Snack			Yes/No	
Dinner			Yes/No	
Other			Yes/No	
	Total Calories Consumed			
	Total Liquid Calories Consumed			
	Total Calories Allowed			

THE OMNI DIET DAILY JOURNAL

Become A Warrior For Your Health! Phase Two-Week Two

DAY THREE

What is my desired outcome for the day? (Why MUST I do this?)

_____

_____

Three Things I am Grateful for Today:

1. _____

2. _____

3. _____

Today's Weight	Hours Slept Last Night	Managed stress ?

On a scale of 1 to 10 rate the following: (1 = poor, 10 = great)			
Mood	Energy	Digestion	Other Symptoms

Write your own mantra. Say it until you believe it.

_____

_____

Choose 5 healthy habits from the list below.

☐ Exercise 1 extra day each week   ☐ Drink fresh green drinks 2X a week

☐ Lift weights at least 2X each week   ☐ Go in the sauna 2X each week

☐ Drink 1 extra glass of water daily   ☐ Write 5 things you're grateful for each morning

☐ Eat 1 extra cup of vegetables daily   ☐ Mentor someone who wants improved health

☐ Write in a food journal every day   ☐ List your daily victories in a victory journal

☐ Find an accountability buddy (AB)   ☐ Review your goals and values

☐ Talk to your AB 2X each week   ☐ Pray/meditate for 5 minutes daily

☐ Do "The Work of Byron Katie": www.thework.com

☐ Post a photo of someone you admire who mirrors your goals

MOTIVATIONAL BLAST:

The sovereign invigorator of the body is exercise, and of all the exercises walking is the best.
— _Thomas Jefferson_

THE OMNI DIET DAILY JOURNAL

If You Fail to Plan, You Plan to Fail. Plan Your Meals for Tomorrow.

DAY FOUR		Date _____	
Time	**Food & Beverages**	**Calories**	**Healthy?**
	Breakfast		Yes/No
	Snack		Yes/No
	Lunch		Yes/No
	Snack		Yes/No
	Dinner		Yes/No
	Other		Yes/No
	Total Calories Consumed		
	Total Liquid Calories Consumed		
	Total Calories Allowed		

THE OMNI DIET DAILY JOURNAL

Become A Warrior For Your Health! Phase Two-Week Two

What is my desired outcome for the day? (Why MUST I do this?)

_____

_____

Three Things I am Grateful for Today:

1. _____

2. _____

3. _____

Today's Weight	Hours Slept Last Night	Managed stress ?

On a scale of 1 to 10 rate the following: (1 = poor, 10 = great)			
Mood	Energy	Digestion	Other Symptoms

Write your own mantra. Say it until you believe it.

_____

_____

Choose 5 healthy habits from the list below.

- ☐ Exercise 1 extra day each week
- ☐ Lift weights at least 2X each week
- ☐ Drink 1 extra glass of water daily
- ☐ Eat 1 extra cup of vegetables daily
- ☐ Write in a food journal every day
- ☐ Find an accountability buddy (AB)
- ☐ Talk to your AB 2X each week
- ☐ Do "The Work of Byron Katie": www.thework.com
- ☐ Post a photo of someone you admire who mirrors your goals
- ☐ Drink fresh green drinks 2X a week
- ☐ Go in the sauna 2X each week
- ☐ Write 5 things you're grateful for each morning
- ☐ Mentor someone who wants improved health
- ☐ List your daily victories in a victory journal
- ☐ Review your goals and values
- ☐ Pray/meditate for 5 minutes daily

MOTIVATIONAL BLAST:

Get Health. No labor, effort nor exercise that can gain it must be grudged.
— Ralph Waldo Emerson

THE OMNI DIET DAILY JOURNAL

If You Fail to Plan, You Plan to Fail. Plan Your Meals for Tomorrow.

| DAY FIVE | | Date _____ | | |

Time	Food & Beverages	Calories	Healthy?
Breakfast			Yes/No
Snack			Yes/No
Lunch			Yes/No
Snack			Yes/No
Dinner			Yes/No
Other			Yes/No
	Total Calories Consumed		
	Total Liquid Calories Consumed		
	Total Calories Allowed		

THE OMNI DIET DAILY JOURNAL

Become A Warrior For Your Health! Phase Two-Week Two

What is my desired outcome for the day? (Why MUST I do this?)

_____

_____

Three Things I am Grateful for Today:

1. _____

2. _____

3. _____

Today's Weight	Hours Slept Last Night	Managed stress ?

On a scale of 1 to 10 rate the following: (1 = poor, 10 = great)			
Mood	Energy	Digestion	Other Symptoms

Write your own mantra. Say it until you believe it.

_____

_____

Choose 5 healthy habits from the list below.

- ☐ Exercise 1 extra day each week
- ☐ Lift weights at least 2X each week
- ☐ Drink 1 extra glass of water daily
- ☐ Eat 1 extra cup of vegetables daily
- ☐ Write in a food journal every day
- ☐ Find an accountability buddy (AB)
- ☐ Talk to your AB 2X each week
- ☐ Drink fresh green drinks 2X a week
- ☐ Go in the sauna 2X each week
- ☐ Write 5 things you're grateful for each morning
- ☐ Mentor someone who wants improved health
- ☐ List your daily victories in a victory journal
- ☐ Review your goals and values
- ☐ Pray/meditate for 5 minutes daily
- ☐ Do "The Work of Byron Katie": www.thework.com
- ☐ Post a photo of someone you admire who mirrors your goals

MOTIVATIONAL BLAST:

You cannot plough a field by turning it over in your mind. — Unknown

THE OMNI DIET DAILY JOURNAL

If You Fail to Plan, You Plan to Fail. Plan Your Meals for Tomorrow.

DAY SIX	Date _____		
Time	**Food & Beverages**	**Calories**	**Healthy?**
Breakfast			Yes/No
Snack			Yes/No
Lunch			Yes/No
Snack			Yes/No
Dinner			Yes/No
Other			Yes/No
	Total Calories Consumed		
	Total Liquid Calories Consumed		
	Total Calories Allowed		

THE OMNI DIET DAILY JOURNAL

Become A Warrior For Your Health! Phase Two-Week Two

DAY SIX

What is my desired outcome for the day? (Why MUST I do this?)

_____

_____

Three Things I am Grateful for Today:

1. _____

2. _____

3. _____

Today's Weight	Hours Slept Last Night	Managed stress ?

On a scale of 1 to 10 rate the following: (1 = poor, 10 = great)			
Mood	Energy	Digestion	Other Symptoms

Write your own mantra. Say it until you believe it.

_____

_____

Choose 5 healthy habits from the list below.

☐ Exercise 1 extra day each week   ☐ Drink fresh green drinks 2X a week

☐ Lift weights at least 2X each week   ☐ Go in the sauna 2X each week

☐ Drink 1 extra glass of water daily   ☐ Write 5 things you're grateful for each morning

☐ Eat 1 extra cup of vegetables daily   ☐ Mentor someone who wants improved health

☐ Write in a food journal every day   ☐ List your daily victories in a victory journal

☐ Find an accountability buddy (AB)   ☐ Review your goals and values

☐ Talk to your AB 2X each week   ☐ Pray/meditate for 5 minutes daily

☐ Do "The Work of Byron Katie": www.thework.com

☐ Post a photo of someone you admire who mirrors your goals

MOTIVATIONAL BLAST:

Nothing lifts me out of a bad mood better than a hard workout on my treadmill. It never fails. To us, exercise is nothing short of a miracle. — Cher

THE OMNI DIET DAILY JOURNAL

If You Fail to Plan, You Plan to Fail. Plan Your Meals for Tomorrow.

	DAY SEVEN	Date _____	
Time	**Food & Beverages**	**Calories**	**Healthy?**
	Breakfast		Yes/No
	Snack		Yes/No
	Lunch		Yes/No
	Snack		Yes/No
	Dinner		Yes/No
	Other		Yes/No
	Total Calories Consumed		
	Total Liquid Calories Consumed		
	Total Calories Allowed		

THE OMNI DIET DAILY JOURNAL

Become A Warrior For Your Health! Phase Two-Week Two

DAY SEVEN

What is my desired outcome for the day? (Why MUST I do this?)

_____

_____

Three Things I am Grateful for Today:

1. _____

2. _____

3. _____

Today's Weight	Hours Slept Last Night	Managed stress ?

On a scale of 1 to 10 rate the following: (1 = poor, 10 = great)			
Mood	Energy	Digestion	Other Symptoms

Write your own mantra. Say it until you believe it.

_____

_____

Choose 5 healthy habits from the list below.

☐ Exercise 1 extra day each week   ☐ Drink fresh green drinks 2X a week

☐ Lift weights at least 2X each week   ☐ Go in the sauna 2X each week

☐ Drink 1 extra glass of water daily   ☐ Write 5 things you're grateful for each morning

☐ Eat 1 extra cup of vegetables daily   ☐ Mentor someone who wants improved health

☐ Write in a food journal every day   ☐ List your daily victories in a victory journal

☐ Find an accountability buddy (AB)   ☐ Review your goals and values

☐ Talk to your AB 2X each week   ☐ Pray/meditate for 5 minutes daily

☐ Do "The Work of Byron Katie": www.thework.com

☐ Post a photo of someone you admire who mirrors your goals

MOTIVATIONAL BLAST:

Lack of activity destroys the good condition of every human being, while movement and methodical physical exercise save it and preserve it. — Plato

THE OMNI DIET DAILY JOURNAL
PHASE TWO-WEEK TWO SUMMARY

	This Week	Goal for Next Week
Weight		
Number of Days I Slept 7 or More Hours		
Number of Days I Exercised at Least 30 Minutes		
Number of Days I Drank My Water Requirement		
Number of Days I Stayed Under My Allowed Calories		
Overall Weekly Energy Level (Low/Average/Good)		

Did I Accomplish My Goals Set This Week? (Circle One)		
Achieved	Over Achieved	Will Try Again!

My struggles this week were:

_____

_____

_____

_____

Ways I can achieve my goals next week:

_____

_____

_____

_____

My biggest accomplishment this week:

_____

_____

_____

Relax Your Way To Better Health

MAKE 90/10 YOUR GOLDEN RULE

If you've carefully followed the program for four weeks now, you should see major changes in how you look and feel. Cravings should be a rare experience, and The Omni Diet is now a way of life! .

I know nobody's perfect, and we don't live in a vacuum. If you have successfully kicked your addiction to sugar, you should now be able to add small treats into your program without feeling guilty. This is a program for life. You can live a full, normal life while still adhering to an eating program that will add to the quality of your life. Here are some ways to expand your eating program to allow for more flexibility while staying on track.

- **90/10 rule:** If you follow the Omni Diet 90% of the time, you can be a bit more relaxed with your food choices 10% of the time. A little extra room is built in so you can enjoy the social aspect of life. At times your choices may be less than optimal due to travel or other circumstances. You should still avoid trigger foods and foods that affect your health (e.g., gluten or dairy).

- **3-bite rule:** If after careful consideration you decide to eat something off plan, follow the three-bite rule we discussed earlier. Most of the pleasure is in the first three bites anyway. So, as you have your three (average size!) bites, be fully present and conscious so you can really concentrate on enjoying the food. Then, after three bites, throw the rest away.

- **Reintroduce small amounts of grains (non gluten) and legumes:** But eat them more like a condiment than a staple - no more than ½ cup, a couple of times each week. And if you feel you don't want them at all, great!

- **When you MUST cheat:** At times you may forget to bring your lunch, or have no time to prepare it. Or you may attend an event that doesn't allow you to bring in food. (Remember, if you are diabetic, lactose intolerant, gluten intolerant, or have special dietary needs, you must be allowed to bring your food with you unless the venue can accommodate your needs.) At amusement parks and parties you may want to relax a little. Just don't be caught off guard. Plan ahead, like this:

  o Decide to eat one non-Omni food. That's not an excuse to eat lousy for the entire day. On average, it takes about three days to feel well and lose your cravings again after only one day of gorging on sugar and fat.

  o Be brutally honest with yourself about your addictions. If you know that you are still vulnerable to relapse, give yourself several more weeks before loosening the reins.

  o Scout out healthy lunch alternatives in your area in advance for the times that you find yourself without your lunch bag.

  o Make the healthiest choices possible from the selection available.

  o When you do make the decision to indulge, make it a conscious decision, and enjoy the moment without guilt. Afterward, be honest about how you feel. Usually you don't feel great. Remember that feeling and you won't be as tempted another time.

  o On the rare occasion that you make an impulsive decision, beating yourself up about it is never helpful. Turn around and get back on track without judgments, criticisms, or anger.

A Plan to Overcome Temptation

EXERCISE

An old expression tells us that "forewarned is forearmed." It's certainly true when it comes to sticking with your healthy eating program in the face of all the temptations you're bound to run into.

The purpose of this exercise is to help you set up a plan so that you will be forearmed in tempting situations.

Take a piece of paper and write down the names of situations where you face temptation, and then jot down ideas for how you will handle them. Select situations that are specific to you, and be precise in how you will prepare.

For example:

DINNER AT IN-LAWS

I will bring a healthy snack so I won't be vulnerable.

I will offer to bring a salad, a healthy dessert, or a side dish so I know there will be something for me to eat.

I will bring a healthy treat to eat with our after-dinner coffee while others are eating dessert.

If they put a dressing with mayonnaise, croutons, or other non-Omni ingredients on the salad, I will ask for my salad without those ingredients, and see if they have a little olive oil and vinegar I can use instead (or bring my own).

I will not drink any alcohol. I'll have water with lemon slices (Or, I will sip on a half-glass of wine filled with ice cubes).

If it's a special occasion (e.g., birthday party), I will have a few bites of cake, but that's all. Or I will stay and sing, but go for a walk until after the cake is eaten.

DINNER OUT

I will eat a healthy snack before going so I won't be starving.

I will try to get others to agree to go to a place where it will be easier to make healthy choices.

I will ask the waiter to remove bread baskets, chips, etc. If others want to eat them, I will know they are on the table but I will try to avoid looking at them, and ask for raw vegetables instead.

I will ask the waitperson about ingredients in dishes and will avoid unhealthy dishes and ask to make healthy substitutions.

I will drink sparkling water or a non-alcoholic, sugar-free beverage. If it's a special occasion I will have one small glass of wine.

I will take home leftovers instead of emptying my plate at one meal.

If it's a special occasion and my companion wants a dessert, I will have one bite only.

Do you get the idea? Now go through this exercise for the situations where you face temptation.

THE OMNI DIET DAILY JOURNAL
PHASE THREE-WEEK ONE

THE OMNI DIET DAILY JOURNAL

If You Fail to Plan, You Plan to Fail. Plan Your Meals for Tomorrow.

Time	DAY ONE Food & Beverages	Date	Calories	Healthy?
	Breakfast			Yes/No
	Snack			Yes/No
	Lunch			Yes/No
	Snack			Yes/No
	Dinner			Yes/No
	Other			Yes/No
	Total Calories Consumed			
	Total Liquid Calories Consumed			
	Total Calories Allowed			

THE OMNI DIET DAILY JOURNAL

Become A Warrior For Your Health! Phase Three-Week One

DAY ONE

What is my desired outcome for the day? (Why MUST I do this?)

_____

_____

Three Things I am Grateful for Today:

1. _____

2. _____

3. _____

Today's Weight	Hours Slept Last Night	Managed stress ?

On a scale of 1 to 10 rate the following: (1 = poor, 10 = great)			
Mood	Energy	Digestion	Other Symptoms

Write your own mantra. Say it until you believe it.

_____

_____

Choose 5 healthy habits from the list below.

☐ Exercise 1 extra day each week   ☐ Drink fresh green drinks 2X a week

☐ Lift weights at least 2X each week   ☐ Go in the sauna 2X each week

☐ Drink 1 extra glass of water daily   ☐ Write 5 things you're grateful for each morning

☐ Eat 1 extra cup of vegetables daily   ☐ Mentor someone who wants improved health

☐ Write in a food journal every day   ☐ List your daily victories in a victory journal

☐ Find an accountability buddy (AB)   ☐ Review your goals and values

☐ Talk to your AB 2X each week   ☐ Pray/meditate for 5 minutes daily

☐ Do "The Work of Byron Katie": www.thework.com

☐ Post a photo of someone you admire who mirrors your goals

MOTIVATIONAL BLAST:

Tension is who you think you should be. Relaxation is who you are." — Chinese Proverb

THE OMNI DIET DAILY JOURNAL

If You Fail to Plan, You Plan to Fail. Plan Your Meals for Tomorrow.

| DAY TWO | Date |

Time	Food & Beverages	Calories	Healthy?
Breakfast			Yes/No
Snack			Yes/No
Lunch			Yes/No
Snack			Yes/No
Dinner			Yes/No
Other			Yes/No
	Total Calories Consumed		
	Total Liquid Calories Consumed		
	Total Calories Allowed		

THE OMNI DIET DAILY JOURNAL
Become A Warrior For Your Health! Phase Three-Week One

DAY TWO

What is my desired outcome for the day? (Why MUST I do this?)

_____

_____

Three Things I am Grateful for Today:

1. _____

2. _____

3. _____

Today's Weight	Hours Slept Last Night	Managed stress ?

On a scale of 1 to 10 rate the following: (1 = poor, 10 = great)			
Mood	Energy	Digestion	Other Symptoms

Write your own mantra. Say it until you believe it.

_____

_____

Choose 5 healthy habits from the list below.

☐ Exercise 1 extra day each week   ☐ Drink fresh green drinks 2X a week

☐ Lift weights at least 2X each week   ☐ Go in the sauna 2X each week

☐ Drink 1 extra glass of water daily   ☐ Write 5 things you're grateful for each morning

☐ Eat 1 extra cup of vegetables daily   ☐ Mentor someone who wants improved health

☐ Write in a food journal every day   ☐ List your daily victories in a victory journal

☐ Find an accountability buddy (AB)   ☐ Review your goals and values

☐ Talk to your AB 2X each week   ☐ Pray/meditate for 5 minutes daily

☐ Do "The Work of Byron Katie": www.thework.com

☐ Post a photo of someone you admire who mirrors your goals

MOTIVATIONAL BLAST:

To wish to be well is a part of becoming well. — Seneca

THE OMNI DIET DAILY JOURNAL

If You Fail to Plan, You Plan to Fail. Plan Your Meals for Tomorrow.

	DAY THREE	Date _____		
Time	**Food & Beverages**		**Calories**	**Healthy?**
Breakfast				Yes/No
Snack				Yes/No
Lunch				Yes/No
Snack				Yes/No
Dinner				Yes/No
Other				Yes/No
	Total Calories Consumed			
	Total Liquid Calories Consumed			
	Total Calories Allowed			

THE OMNI DIET DAILY JOURNAL

Become A Warrior For Your Health! Phase Three-Week One

What is my desired outcome for the day? (Why MUST I do this?)

_____

_____

Three Things I am Grateful for Today:

1. _____

2. _____

3. _____

Today's Weight	Hours Slept Last Night	Managed stress ?

On a scale of 1 to 10 rate the following: (1 = poor, 10 = great)			
Mood	Energy	Digestion	Other Symptoms

Write your own mantra. Say it until you believe it.

_____

_____

Choose 5 healthy habits from the list below.

☐ Exercise 1 extra day each week   ☐ Drink fresh green drinks 2X a week

☐ Lift weights at least 2X each week   ☐ Go in the sauna 2X each week

☐ Drink 1 extra glass of water daily   ☐ Write 5 things you're grateful for each morning

☐ Eat 1 extra cup of vegetables daily   ☐ Mentor someone who wants improved health

☐ Write in a food journal every day   ☐ List your daily victories in a victory journal

☐ Find an accountability buddy (AB)   ☐ Review your goals and values

☐ Talk to your AB 2X each week   ☐ Pray/meditate for 5 minutes daily

☐ Do "The Work of Byron Katie": www.thework.com

☐ Post a photo of someone you admire who mirrors your goals

MOTIVATIONAL BLAST:

He who takes medicine and neglects his diet wastes the skill of his doctors.
— Chinese Proverb

THE OMNI DIET DAILY JOURNAL

If You Fail to Plan, You Plan to Fail. Plan Your Meals for Tomorrow.

DAY FOUR		Date _____	
Time	**Food & Beverages**	**Calories**	**Healthy?**
Breakfast			Yes/No
Snack			Yes/No
Lunch			Yes/No
Snack			Yes/No
Dinner			Yes/No
Other			Yes/No
	Total Calories Consumed		
	Total Liquid Calories Consumed		
	Total Calories Allowed		

THE OMNI DIET DAILY JOURNAL

Become A Warrior For Your Health! Phase Three-Week One

DAY FOUR

What is my desired outcome for the day? (Why MUST I do this?)

_____

_____

Three Things I am Grateful for Today:

1. _____

2. _____

3. _____

Today's Weight	Hours Slept Last Night	Managed stress ?

On a scale of 1 to 10 rate the following: (1 = poor, 10 = great)			
Mood	Energy	Digestion	Other Symptoms

Write your own mantra. Say it until you believe it.

_____

_____

Choose 5 healthy habits from the list below.

☐ Exercise 1 extra day each week   ☐ Drink fresh green drinks 2X a week

☐ Lift weights at least 2X each week   ☐ Go in the sauna 2X each week

☐ Drink 1 extra glass of water daily   ☐ Write 5 things you're grateful for each morning

☐ Eat 1 extra cup of vegetables daily   ☐ Mentor someone who wants improved health

☐ Write in a food journal every day   ☐ List your daily victories in a victory journal

☐ Find an accountability buddy (AB)   ☐ Review your goals and values

☐ Talk to your AB 2X each week   ☐ Pray/meditate for 5 minutes daily

☐ Do "The Work of Byron Katie": www.thework.com

☐ Post a photo of someone you admire who mirrors your goals

MOTIVATIONAL BLAST:

Those who have no time for healthy eating will sooner or later have to find time for illness.
— Edward Stanley

THE OMNI DIET DAILY JOURNAL

If You Fail to Plan, You Plan to Fail. Plan Your Meals for Tomorrow.

DAY FIVE	Date _____

Time	Food & Beverages	Calories	Healthy?
Breakfast			Yes/No
Snack			Yes/No
Lunch			Yes/No
Snack			Yes/No
Dinner			Yes/No
Other			Yes/No
	Total Calories Consumed		
	Total Liquid Calories Consumed		
	Total Calories Allowed		

THE OMNI DIET DAILY JOURNAL

Become A Warrior For Your Health! Phase Three-Week One

DAY FIVE

What is my desired outcome for the day? (Why MUST I do this?)

_____

_____

Three Things I am Grateful for Today:

1. _____

2. _____

3. _____

Today's Weight	Hours Slept Last Night	Managed stress ?

On a scale of 1 to 10 rate the following: (1 = poor, 10 = great)			
Mood	Energy	Digestion	Other Symptoms

Write your own mantra. Say it until you believe it.

_____

_____

Choose 5 healthy habits from the list below.

☐ Exercise 1 extra day each week

☐ Lift weights at least 2X each week

☐ Drink 1 extra glass of water daily

☐ Eat 1 extra cup of vegetables daily

☐ Write in a food journal every day

☐ Find an accountability buddy (AB)

☐ Talk to your AB 2X each week

☐ Drink fresh green drinks 2X a week

☐ Go in the sauna 2X each week

☐ Write 5 things you're grateful for each morning

☐ Mentor someone who wants improved health

☐ List your daily victories in a victory journal

☐ Review your goals and values

☐ Pray/meditate for 5 minutes daily

☐ Do "The Work of Byron Katie": www.thework.com

☐ Post a photo of someone you admire who mirrors your goals

MOTIVATIONAL BLAST:

At first glance it may appear too hard. Look again. Always look again.
— _Mary Anne Rodmacher_

THE OMNI DIET DAILY JOURNAL

If You Fail to Plan, You Plan to Fail. Plan Your Meals for Tomorrow.

Time	Food & Beverages	Calories	Healthy?
	DAY SIX Date _____		
	Breakfast		Yes/No
	Snack		Yes/No
	Lunch		Yes/No
	Snack		Yes/No
	Dinner		Yes/No
	Other		Yes/No
	Total Calories Consumed		
	Total Liquid Calories Consumed		
	Total Calories Allowed		

THE OMNI DIET DAILY JOURNAL

Become A Warrior For Your Health! Phase Three-Week One

What is my desired outcome for the day? (Why MUST I do this?)

_____

_____

Three Things I am Grateful for Today:

1. _____

2. _____

3. _____

Today's Weight	Hours Slept Last Night	Managed stress ?

On a scale of 1 to 10 rate the following: (1 = poor, 10 = great)			
Mood	Energy	Digestion	Other Symptoms

Write your own mantra. Say it until you believe it.

_____

_____

Choose 5 healthy habits from the list below.

☐ Exercise 1 extra day each week   ☐ Drink fresh green drinks 2X a week

☐ Lift weights at least 2X each week   ☐ Go in the sauna 2X each week

☐ Drink 1 extra glass of water daily   ☐ Write 5 things you're grateful for each morning

☐ Eat 1 extra cup of vegetables daily   ☐ Mentor someone who wants improved health

☐ Write in a food journal every day   ☐ List your daily victories in a victory journal

☐ Find an accountability buddy (AB)   ☐ Review your goals and values

☐ Talk to your AB 2X each week   ☐ Pray/meditate for 5 minutes daily

☐ Do "The Work of Byron Katie": www.thework.com

☐ Post a photo of someone you admire who mirrors your goals

MOTIVATIONAL BLAST:

The more you eat, the less flavor; the less you eat, the more flavor. — _Chinese Proverb_

THE OMNI DIET DAILY JOURNAL

If You Fail to Plan, You Plan to Fail. Plan Your Meals for Tomorrow.

| | DAY SEVEN | Date _____ | | |

Time	Food & Beverages		Calories	Healthy?
Breakfast				Yes/No
Snack				Yes/No
Lunch				Yes/No
Snack				Yes/No
Dinner				Yes/No
Other				Yes/No
	Total Calories Consumed			
	Total Liquid Calories Consumed			
	Total Calories Allowed			

THE OMNI DIET DAILY JOURNAL

Become A Warrior For Your Health! Phase Three-Week One

What is my desired outcome for the day? (Why MUST I do this?)

_____

_____

Three Things I am Grateful for Today:

1. _____

2. _____

3. _____

Today's Weight	Hours Slept Last Night	Managed stress ?

On a scale of 1 to 10 rate the following: (1 = poor, 10 = great)			
Mood	Energy	Digestion	Other Symptoms

Write your own mantra. Say it until you believe it.

_____

_____

Choose 5 healthy habits from the list below.

☐ Exercise 1 extra day each week   ☐ Drink fresh green drinks 2X a week

☐ Lift weights at least 2X each week   ☐ Go in the sauna 2X each week

☐ Drink 1 extra glass of water daily   ☐ Write 5 things you're grateful for each morning

☐ Eat 1 extra cup of vegetables daily   ☐ Mentor someone who wants improved health

☐ Write in a food journal every day   ☐ List your daily victories in a victory journal

☐ Find an accountability buddy (AB)   ☐ Review your goals and values

☐ Talk to your AB 2X each week   ☐ Pray/meditate for 5 minutes daily

☐ Do "The Work of Byron Katie": www.thework.com

☐ Post a photo of someone you admire who mirrors your goals

MOTIVATIONAL BLAST:

Nothing is impossible, the word itself says "I'm possible"! — Audrey Hepburn

THE OMNI DIET DAILY JOURNAL
PHASE THREE - WEEK ONE SUMMARY

	This Week	*Goal for Next Week*
Weight		
Number of Days I Slept 7 or More Hours		
Number of Days I Exercised at Least 30 Minutes		
Number of Days I Drank My Water Requirement		
Number of Days I Stayed Under My Allowed Calories		
Overall Weekly Energy Level (Low/Average/Good)		

Did I accomplish my goals set last week? (Circle One)		
Achieved	Over Achieved	Will Try Again!

My struggles this week were:

_____

_____

_____

_____

Ways I can achieve my goals next week:

_____

_____

_____

_____

My biggest accomplishment this week:

_____

_____

_____

Relax Your Way To Better Health

BETTER SLEEP AND LESS STRESS

All the results of your hard work and healthy eating can be derailed by poor sleep and stress.

Why Sleep Is Important

Sleep is a cornerstone of long-term brain health and vibrant energy. It also plays a surprising part in weight control. Many studies have shown that chronic failure to get enough sleep increases the risk of being overweight or obese. You should get at least seven hours of sleep per night.

- Sleep restriction lowers levels of leptin, the hormone that tells you to stop eating when you're full. When leptin is low, your brain receives the message that you should eat more, even if your body doesn't actually need more calories.

- Not getting enough sleep increases levels of the hormone ghrelin, which promotes appetite. And it increases levels of orexin, a neurotransmitter that increases food cravings.

- Being overtired interrupts healthy glucose metabolism, making your body more resistant to insulin. Over time, the increased demand on the pancreas from insulin resistance can compromise beta-cell function and lead to type 2 diabetes.

- Lack of sleep is linked to high blood pressure, heart attack, and increased risk of car accidents, depression, and substance abuse. You don't need scientific research to tell you that when people are exhausted they become forgetful, inattentive, and irritable.

- When you feel refreshed and rested, you feel energized, think clearly, and are much more likely to make smart choices about eating and exercising.

Why You Must Keep Stress Under Control

Chronic stress causes damaging chemical and hormonal reactions. Cutting down the stress in your life—and developing good coping skills to help you deal with stresses that you can't control—is good for your health and your weight.

- When your body constantly produces too much of the stress hormone cortisol, it triggers increases in blood sugar and belly fat as well as changes in your metabolism.

- Another hormone, norepinephrine, can cause blood pressure to go up and can aggravate attention deficit disorder.

- SPECT scans of the brain of someone who's meditating compared with scans of someone who's stressed show dramatic differences in blood flow and neurotransmitter activity.

- Chronic stress lowers brain activity, which increases your vulnerability to depression, anxiety, impulsiveness, and illness.

- It contributes to weight gain and the buildup of belly fat, which is especially lethal because it surrounds and impacts the health of vital organs in the core of your body.

Steps to Improve Sleep and Reduce Stress

EXERCISE

In The Omni Diet I list and explain a number of very effective ways to improve your sleep and reduce your stress. For this week's exercise, select a few of these suggestions and put them to work. See if it makes a difference.

Improve Your Sleep

Check off 3 of the following 12 steps you can take to improve your sleep, and work with them for a week.

☐ Keep your sleeping area dark
☐ Relax with guided meditation, soothing music
☐ Go to bed and get up on a regular schedule
☐ Use a white noise machine
☐ Power down computers and all electronic devices
☐ Have a soothing drink: chamomile tea, cocoa, etc
☐ Take a soothing bath
☐ Make love (orgasm promotes better sleep)
☐ Block out noise
☐ Get up for a short time, then go back to bed
☐ Avoid strenuous exercise 3 hours before bedtime
☐ Write down racing thoughts and clear your mind

Reduce Stress

Check off 3 of the following 12 steps you can take to improve your sleep, and work with them for a week.

☐ Engage in moderate exercise
☐ Use hypnosis (especially self-hypnosis

- [ ] Write down stressors and possible solutions
- [ ] Pray and meditate
- [ ] Start saying "No" to demands
- [ ] Kill the ANTs (automatic negative thoughts)
- [ ] Surround yourself with positive, happy people
- [ ] Write down 5 things you're grateful for each day
- [ ] Find shortcuts that simplify your life
- [ ] Say an incantation (affirmation) until you feel it
- [ ] Practice relaxation skills
- [ ] Reach out to others for love, support, connection

In coming weeks experiment with other items on each of the lists. Find the best program for you that reduces your stress and helps you sleep soundly.

THE OMNI DIET DAILY JOURNAL
PHASE THREE-WEEK TWO

THE OMNI DIET DAILY JOURNAL

If You Fail to Plan, You Plan to Fail. Plan Your Meals for Tomorrow.

Time	DAY ONE — Food & Beverages	Date _____ Calories	Healthy?
	Breakfast		Yes/No
	Snack		Yes/No
	Lunch		Yes/No
	Snack		Yes/No
	Dinner		Yes/No
	Other		Yes/No
	Total Calories Consumed		
	Total Liquid Calories Consumed		
	Total Calories Allowed		

THE OMNI DIET DAILY JOURNAL

Become A Warrior For Your Health! Phase Three-Week Three

DAY ONE

What is my desired outcome for the day? (Why MUST I do this?)

_____

_____

Three Things I am Grateful for Today:

1. _____

2. _____

3. _____

Today's Weight	Hours Slept Last Night	Managed stress ?

On a scale of 1 to 10 rate the following: (1 = poor, 10 = great)			
Mood	Energy	Digestion	Other Symptoms

Write your own mantra. Say it until you believe it.

_____

_____

Choose 5 healthy habits from the list below.

☐ Exercise 1 extra day each week   ☐ Drink fresh green drinks 2X a week

☐ Lift weights at least 2X each week   ☐ Go in the sauna 2X each week

☐ Drink 1 extra glass of water daily   ☐ Write 5 things you're grateful for each morning

☐ Eat 1 extra cup of vegetables daily   ☐ Mentor someone who wants improved health

☐ Write in a food journal every day   ☐ List your daily victories in a victory journal

☐ Find an accountability buddy (AB)   ☐ Review your goals and values

☐ Talk to your AB 2X each week   ☐ Pray/meditate for 5 minutes daily

☐ Do "The Work of Byron Katie": www.thework.com

☐ Post a photo of someone you admire who mirrors your goals

MOTIVATIONAL BLAST:

The doctor of the future will no longer treat the human frame with drugs, but rather will cure and prevent disease with nutrition. — _Thomas Edison_

THE OMNI DIET DAILY JOURNAL

If You Fail to Plan, You Plan to Fail. Plan Your Meals for Tomorrow.

DAY TWO	Date _____

Time	Food & Beverages	Calories	Healthy?
Breakfast			Yes/No
Snack			Yes/No
Lunch			Yes/No
Snack			Yes/No
Dinner			Yes/No
Other			Yes/No
	Total Calories Consumed		
	Total Liquid Calories Consumed		
	Total Calories Allowed		

THE OMNI DIET DAILY JOURNAL

Become A Warrior For Your Health! Phase Three-Week Three

DAY TWO

What is my desired outcome for the day? (Why MUST I do this?)

_____

_____

Three Things I am Grateful for Today:

1. _____

2. _____

3. _____

Today's Weight	Hours Slept Last Night	Managed stress ?

On a scale of 1 to 10 rate the following: (1 = poor, 10 = great)			
Mood	Energy	Digestion	Other Symptoms

Write your own mantra. Say it until you believe it.

_____

_____

Choose 5 healthy habits from the list below.

☐ Exercise 1 extra day each week   ☐ Drink fresh green drinks 2X a week

☐ Lift weights at least 2X each week   ☐ Go in the sauna 2X each week

☐ Drink 1 extra glass of water daily   ☐ Write 5 things you're grateful for each morning

☐ Eat 1 extra cup of vegetables daily   ☐ Mentor someone who wants improved health

☐ Write in a food journal every day   ☐ List your daily victories in a victory journal

☐ Find an accountability buddy (AB)   ☐ Review your goals and values

☐ Talk to your AB 2X each week   ☐ Pray/meditate for 5 minutes daily

☐ Do "The Work of Byron Katie": www.thework.com

☐ Post a photo of someone you admire who mirrors your goals

MOTIVATIONAL BLAST:

A good laugh and a long sleep are the best cures in the doctor's book. — _Irish Proverb_

THE OMNI DIET DAILY JOURNAL

If You Fail to Plan, You Plan to Fail. Plan Your Meals for Tomorrow.

DAY THREE		Date _____		
Time	**Food & Beverages**		**Calories**	**Healthy?**
	Breakfast			Yes/No
	Snack			Yes/No
	Lunch			Yes/No
	Snack			Yes/No
	Dinner			Yes/No
	Other			Yes/No
	Total Calories Consumed			
	Total Liquid Calories Consumed			
	Total Calories Allowed			

THE OMNI DIET DAILY JOURNAL

Become A Warrior For Your Health! Phase Three-Week Three

DAY THREE

What is my desired outcome for the day? (Why MUST I do this?)

_____

_____

Three Things I am Grateful for Today:

1. _____

2. _____

3. _____

Today's Weight	Hours Slept Last Night	Managed stress ?

On a scale of 1 to 10 rate the following: (1 = poor, 10 = great)			
Mood	Energy	Digestion	Other Symptoms

Write your own mantra. Say it until you believe it.

_____

_____

Choose 5 healthy habits from the list below.

☐ Exercise 1 extra day each week   ☐ Drink fresh green drinks 2X a week

☐ Lift weights at least 2X each week   ☐ Go in the sauna 2X each week

☐ Drink 1 extra glass of water daily   ☐ Write 5 things you're grateful for each morning

☐ Eat 1 extra cup of vegetables daily   ☐ Mentor someone who wants improved health

☐ Write in a food journal every day   ☐ List your daily victories in a victory journal

☐ Find an accountability buddy (AB)   ☐ Review your goals and values

☐ Talk to your AB 2X each week   ☐ Pray/meditate for 5 minutes daily

☐ Do "The Work of Byron Katie": www.thework.com

☐ Post a photo of someone you admire who mirrors your goals

MOTIVATIONAL BLAST:

People who laugh actually live longer than those who don't laugh. Few persons realize that health actually varies according to the amount of laughter. — James J. Walsh

THE OMNI DIET DAILY JOURNAL

If You Fail to Plan, You Plan to Fail. Plan Your Meals for Tomorrow.

	DAY FOUR	Date		
Time	**Food & Beverages**		**Calories**	**Healthy?**
	Breakfast			Yes/No
	Snack			Yes/No
	Lunch			Yes/No
	Snack			Yes/No
	Dinner			Yes/No
	Other			Yes/No
	Total Calories Consumed			
	Total Liquid Calories Consumed			
	Total Calories Allowed			

THE OMNI DIET DAILY JOURNAL

Become A Warrior For Your Health! Phase Three-Week Three

DAY FOUR

What is my desired outcome for the day? (Why MUST I do this?)

_____

_____

Three Things I am Grateful for Today:

1. _____

2. _____

3. _____

Today's Weight	Hours Slept Last Night	Managed stress ?

On a scale of 1 to 10 rate the following: (1 = poor, 10 = great)			
Mood	Energy	Digestion	Other Symptoms

Write your own mantra. Say it until you believe it.

_____

_____

Choose 5 healthy habits from the list below.

☐ Exercise 1 extra day each week   ☐ Drink fresh green drinks 2X a week

☐ Lift weights at least 2X each week   ☐ Go in the sauna 2X each week

☐ Drink 1 extra glass of water daily   ☐ Write 5 things you're grateful for each morning

☐ Eat 1 extra cup of vegetables daily   ☐ Mentor someone who wants improved health

☐ Write in a food journal every day   ☐ List your daily victories in a victory journal

☐ Find an accountability buddy (AB)   ☐ Review your goals and values

☐ Talk to your AB 2X each week   ☐ Pray/meditate for 5 minutes daily

☐ Do "The Work of Byron Katie": www.thework.com

☐ Post a photo of someone you admire who mirrors your goals

MOTIVATIONAL BLAST:

Prevention is better than cure. — Desiderius Erasmus

THE OMNI DIET DAILY JOURNAL

If You Fail to Plan, You Plan to Fail. Plan Your Meals for Tomorrow.

Time	Food & Beverages	Calories	Healthy?
DAY FIVE		Date _____	
	Breakfast		Yes/No
	Snack		Yes/No
	Lunch		Yes/No
	Snack		Yes/No
	Dinner		Yes/No
	Other		Yes/No
	Total Calories Consumed		
	Total Liquid Calories Consumed		
	Total Calories Allowed		

THE OMNI DIET DAILY JOURNAL

Become A Warrior For Your Health! Phase Three-Week Three

What is my desired outcome for the day? (Why MUST I do this?)

_____

_____

Three Things I am Grateful for Today:

1. _____

2. _____

3. _____

Today's Weight	Hours Slept Last Night	Managed stress ?

On a scale of 1 to 10 rate the following: (1 = poor, 10 = great)			
Mood	Energy	Digestion	Other Symptoms

Write your own mantra. Say it until you believe it.

_____

_____

Choose 5 healthy habits from the list below.

- ☐ Exercise 1 extra day each week
- ☐ Lift weights at least 2X each week
- ☐ Drink 1 extra glass of water daily
- ☐ Eat 1 extra cup of vegetables daily
- ☐ Write in a food journal every day
- ☐ Find an accountability buddy (AB)
- ☐ Talk to your AB 2X each week
- ☐ Do "The Work of Byron Katie": www.thework.com
- ☐ Post a photo of someone you admire who mirrors your goals
- ☐ Drink fresh green drinks 2X a week
- ☐ Go in the sauna 2X each week
- ☐ Write 5 things you're grateful for each morning
- ☐ Mentor someone who wants improved health
- ☐ List your daily victories in a victory journal
- ☐ Review your goals and values
- ☐ Pray/meditate for 5 minutes daily

MOTIVATIONAL BLAST:

I've learned that no matter what happens, or how bad it seems today, life does go on, and it will be better tomorrow. — Maya Angelou

THE OMNI DIET DAILY JOURNAL

If You Fail to Plan, You Plan to Fail. Plan Your Meals for Tomorrow.

	DAY SIX	Date _____		
Time	**Food & Beverages**		**Calories**	**Healthy?**
Breakfast				Yes/No
Snack				Yes/No
Lunch				Yes/No
Snack				Yes/No
Dinner				Yes/No
Other				Yes/No
	Total Calories Consumed			
	Total Liquid Calories Consumed			
	Total Calories Allowed			

THE OMNI DIET DAILY JOURNAL

Become A Warrior For Your Health! Phase Three-Week Three

DAY SIX

What is my desired outcome for the day? (Why MUST I do this?)

_____

_____

Three Things I am Grateful for Today:

1. _____

2. _____

3. _____

Today's Weight	Hours Slept Last Night	Managed stress ?

On a scale of 1 to 10 rate the following: (1 = poor, 10 = great)			
Mood	Energy	Digestion	Other Symptoms

Write your own mantra. Say it until you believe it.

_____

_____

Choose 5 healthy habits from the list below.

☐ Exercise 1 extra day each week   ☐ Drink fresh green drinks 2X a week

☐ Lift weights at least 2X each week   ☐ Go in the sauna 2X each week

☐ Drink 1 extra glass of water daily   ☐ Write 5 things you're grateful for each morning

☐ Eat 1 extra cup of vegetables daily   ☐ Mentor someone who wants improved health

☐ Write in a food journal every day   ☐ List your daily victories in a victory journal

☐ Find an accountability buddy (AB)   ☐ Review your goals and values

☐ Talk to your AB 2X each week   ☐ Pray/meditate for 5 minutes daily

☐ Do "The Work of Byron Katie": www.thework.com

☐ Post a photo of someone you admire who mirrors your goals

MOTIVATIONAL BLAST:

You've got to say, I think that if I keep working at this and want it badly enough I can have it. It's called perseverance. — Lee Iacocca

THE OMNI DIET DAILY JOURNAL

If You Fail to Plan, You Plan to Fail. Plan Your Meals for Tomorrow.

Time	Food & Beverages	Calories	Healthy?
DAY SEVEN		Date _____	
Breakfast			Yes/No
Snack			Yes/No
Lunch			Yes/No
Snack			Yes/No
Dinner			Yes/No
Other			Yes/No
	Total Calories Consumed		
	Total Liquid Calories Consumed		
	Total Calories Allowed		

THE OMNI DIET DAILY JOURNAL

Become A Warrior For Your Health! Phase Three-Week Three

DAY SEVEN

What is my desired outcome for the day? (Why MUST I do this?)

_____

_____

Three Things I am Grateful for Today:

1. _____

2. _____

3. _____

Today's Weight	Hours Slept Last Night	Managed stress ?

On a scale of 1 to 10 rate the following: (1 = poor, 10 = great)			
Mood	Energy	Digestion	Other Symptoms

Write your own mantra. Say it until you believe it.

_____

_____

Choose 5 healthy habits from the list below.

☐ Exercise 1 extra day each week   ☐ Drink fresh green drinks 2X a week

☐ Lift weights at least 2X each week   ☐ Go in the sauna 2X each week

☐ Drink 1 extra glass of water daily   ☐ Write 5 things you're grateful for each morning

☐ Eat 1 extra cup of vegetables daily   ☐ Mentor someone who wants improved health

☐ Write in a food journal every day   ☐ List your daily victories in a victory journal

☐ Find an accountability buddy (AB)   ☐ Review your goals and values

☐ Talk to your AB 2X each week   ☐ Pray/meditate for 5 minutes daily

☐ Do "The Work of Byron Katie": www.thework.com

☐ Post a photo of someone you admire who mirrors your goals

MOTIVATIONAL BLAST:

There is no passion to be found in playing small—in settling for a life that is less than the one you are capable of living. — Nelson Mandela

THE OMNI DIET DAILY JOURNAL
PHASE THREE-WEEK TWO SUMMARY

	This Week	*Goal for Next Week*
Weight		
Number of Days I Slept 7 or More Hours		
Number of Days I Exercised at Least 30 Minutes		
Number of Days I Drank My Water Requirement		
Number of Days I Stayed Under My Allowed Calories		
Overall Weekly Energy Level (Low/Average/Good)		

Did I Accomplish My Goals Set This Week? (Circle One)

Achieved	Over Achieved	Will Try Again!

My struggles this week were:

_____

_____

_____

_____

Ways I can achieve my goals next week:

_____

_____

_____

_____

My biggest accomplishment this week:

_____

_____

_____